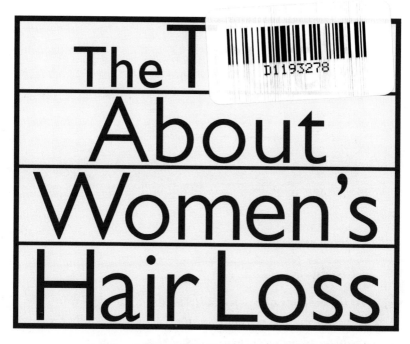

The Truth About Women's Hair Loss

What *Really* Works for Treating and Preventing Thinning Hair

SPENCER DAVID KOBREN

Host of the Nationally Syndicated Radio Program "The Bald Truth"

Foreword by Angela M. Christiano, Ph.D.

CB

CONTEMPORARY BOOKS

Library of Congress Cataloging-in-Publication Data

Kobren, Spencer David.
    The truth about women's hair loss : what really works for treating and
    preventing thinning hair / Spencer David Kobren ; foreword by Angela
    Christiano.
        p.   cm.
    Includes index.
    ISBN 0-8092-2488-7
    1. Baldness.   2. Women—Health and hygiene.   I. Title.
    RL155.K634   2000
    616.5'46—dc21   99-39201
                                                                         CIP

*To the millions of women suffering from hair loss who
deserve so much more respect than they've been given by the
medical, pharmaceutical, and hair loss industries.*

Cover design by Mary Lockwood
Interior design by Amy Yu Ng

Published by Contemporary Books
A division of NTC/Contemporary Publishing Group, Inc.
4255 West Touhy Avenue, Lincolnwood (Chicago), Illinois 60712-1975 U.S.A.
Printed in the United States of America
International Standard Book Number: 0-8092-2488-7
00 01 02 03 04 05 ML 19 18 17 16 15 14 13 12 11 10 9 8 7 6 5 4 3 2

Contents

Foreword

by Angela M. Christiano, Ph.D.

*In the fall of 1997, Dr. Christiano discovered "the hairless
gene," the first gene linked to hair loss. She continues her
search for other hair loss genes.*

In 3,000 B.C., history records the first reference to a woman dealing with the madness of hair loss in the story of Queen Mother
Ses of Egypt, who suffered from "falling hair." In their wisdom,
her doctors prescribed a prayer and a prescription. The prayer is
recited as follows:

> O! Shining One, Thou who hoverest above!
> O! Xare! O Disco of the Sun!
> O Protector of the Divine!

The invocation was followed by a tonic, taken orally, which
consisted of a delicate elixir of "a bolus of iron, red lead, onions,
alabaster, and honey."

Nearly five thousand years have passed since Queen Ses's
desperate quest for a cure to her hair loss. The success of this
treatment was not recorded, and the Queen and her dermatologists have long since faded into history. But for the millions of us
through the centuries who have tried similar unfounded hair loss

remedies, concoctions, and mystical potions, this story reaches across time.

In the same five thousand years, we have made extraordinary progress as a civilization—we have eradicated viruses, built bridges, erected skyscrapers, harnessed electricity, transplanted organs from one person to another, and sent people orbiting into the cosmos and now into the frontiers of cyberspace. And yet the mysteries of a structure so tiny and humble as the human hair follicle continue to elude us.

While scientific research into the basis of hair loss is finally gaining momentum as we approach the millennium, what are women supposed to do in the meantime? "Just sit back and don't stress out about it," our physicians so often advise. Do nothing except watch your hair slowly disappear down the drain— literally.

Hair loss is all too familiar to many women, and is bound to touch all of our lives in some way. Sometimes it can come to us in the form of common androgenetic alopecia, in which the hair part gets wider and wider and hair slowly vanishes as we age, stealing with it our youth and beauty. It may come to us in the form of hair shedding after pregnancy, the insidious round bald patches of alopecia areata, the traction alopecia as a result of elaborate hairstyles, or the sadness of even temporary hair loss following chemotherapy.

Queen Ses and later the Bible tell us that "the long hair of a woman is her glory" (1 Cor. 11.2–16). Women react to hair loss by feeling the obvious pain over the loss of control and the fading of beauty, followed by feelings of guilt and foolishness over feeling so vain. We try to be strong and tell ourselves that we will like ourselves with or without hair and that our partners will surely love us when we're bald.

But deep in the darkest of hours, we acknowledge that hair loss quietly robs us of our souls and our self-esteem—the essence of our very selves.

Hair loss knocked on my door almost four years ago, at a very stressful time in my life. I had just turned thirty, divorced my husband, moved to Manhattan, and started my own laboratory at Columbia University. Six months later, while I was having my hair highlighted, my stylist noticed three bald spots on the back of my head—such was my introduction to the madness that is alopecia areata.

When the Unexpected knocks at your door, you can either slam the door in its face, or invite it in and throw something in the oven.

I chose to start cooking.

What followed for me has been an amazing journey into the land of the "follicularly challenged." Had my hair not fallen out, I would not have redirected my research program into the genetics of alopecia, discovered the first gene linked to hair loss, or be writing this today. Nor would I have met the many colleagues I now call friends, especially the author of this book.

The Truth About Women's Hair Loss is Spencer David Kobren's second book about world of hair. The first was his groundbreaking book, *The Bald Truth.* In response to his own unexpected hair loss in his twenties, Spencer, like me, chose to devote his life to a singular mission: to tell the truth about hair loss treatments and to prevent consumers from ever again being taken advantage of by unscrupulous snake-oil peddlers. Hair loss sufferers are extremely vulnerable to the sleek sales tactics of these people who are no better than criminals. In this book, designed especially for women and written in Kobren's inimitable frank and informative yet softly humorous style, he once again sets out to set the record straight and put the hair loss charlatans out of business.

He also provides a complete, no-nonsense guide to the arsenal of traditional and alternative natural medical approaches to hair loss to help women tailor their own treatment programs to their needs. Most importantly, Kobren reminds us to seek medical advice and helps us determine how best to find those who are qualified and compassionate.

While we are still temporarily stuck in a world of gender-based clinical drug trials targeted at men and further insulted by the fact that one of the major kinds of hair loss routinely affecting women—androgenetic alopecia—is still called "male pattern baldness," *The Truth About Women's Hair Loss* provides us with the tools we need to successfully navigate through the maze of hair loss treatments.

Until the day comes when we can retire alopecia, due to the success of modern genetic medicine, Spencer David Kobren is our voice of truth in the madness of hair loss and the hair loss industry.

Angela M. Christiano, Ph.D.
Assistant Professor of
Dermatology and Genetics and
Development
Columbia University
College of Physicians and
Surgeons
May 1999

Acknowledgments

This book has been a continuation of the work I began a number of years ago, which led to my first book, *The Bald Truth*, and then to my nationally syndicated radio program of the same name. None of this would have been possible without the tremendous support of my family, friends, and colleagues, without whom I would be one miserable, frustrated, angry consumer/patient advocate.

My dear friend Patricia Lynn Johnson once remarked that I had taken a hair obsession and turned it into a career. I am proud to admit that she's right, and I wish we lived in a world in which a guy like me wasn't needed. I do what I do because I have been (and continue to be) in the same boat as those I work to inform, guide, and support. I didn't plan to do this. It just evolved, and the longer I fight for the rights of my hair loss brothers and sisters, the more obvious it becomes that *every* medical specialty needs advocates and watchdogs, and all people in the world need to be as educated as possible about their health and healing

THE TRUTH ABOUT WOMEN'S HAIR LOSS

options in order to survive, not only the conditions that may befall them, but also the very systems that are in place purportedly to help them.

My deepest thanks to Dr. Angela Christiano, who gave so generously of her time and continues to do so in support of my work; to Dr. Robert M. Bernstein, Dr. William Rassman, David Black, Dr. Ron Shapiro, Dr. Paul Rose, Dr. Ken Washenik, Dr. Marty Sawaya, Dr. O'Tar Norwood, Dr. Bernard Nusbaum, Dr. Barry Sears, Dr. Joe Greco, and the other amazing doctors and researchers who have been of such enormous assistance and who are listed in the Resource Guide at the end of this book.

Thank you, Sandra Stein, for your candid, honest look behind the scenes of the hair transplant world.

Special thanks to my radio producer and friend, Peter Bartholomew, and to the dedicated radio crew, including Dennis Cattlett, Tony Dee, and Brian Dee.

Thanks to Farrel Manne who designed The Bald Truth website and who has supported my efforts from the very beginning; to my lifelong buddy Dan Paige for keeping me laughing; to Rafael Rafaelli III for his continuing wise counsel; to Orhan Secilmis for being Orhan; to Sue Paige, Kathleen Brannen, Barbara Brody, Craig Brody, Janet Firth, Joe Gisondi, Adrian Ball, Ben McGlinn, Lilian Balzana, Brad Brooks, Neil a.k.a. Ross, Izzy, Betty Allen, Sandy Lebowitz, Jeff Barton, Richard McRae, Hiram Wilson, Jesse O'Kane, Don Randall, Brian Klosenski, Brian Taylor, Nancy Thompson, Marcus Braxton, and all those who have shared their experiences, stories, and questions with me via letters, phone calls, and E-mail and during the call-in portion of my radio program.

A very special thanks to consumer advocate pioneer Ralph Nader and his hard-working staff in Washington, D.C.

My father, Jack, my brother, Alan, and my late mother, Doris, have my deepest gratitude.

Thank you to my agent, Regula Noetzli, and my editor at Contemporary Books, Judith McCarthy, for their commitment to this book and the patient advocacy behind it. Thanks, also, to copyeditor Sarah Lane and assistant project editor Kristy Grant.

And, finally, tremendous thanks to journalist and author Nina L. Diamond for her continued editorial and publishing guidance and for once again helping me to bring the words out of my head and onto the page.

Author's Note

The day that I realized that I was losing my hair was one of the most frightening, upsetting, and confusing days of my life.

I was only twenty-two at the time, and the last thing on my mind was contending with hair loss. I had just gotten over my recurring teenage acne breakouts when I was suddenly confronted with hair loss I didn't think I'd have to deal with until I was middle-aged, if ever.

It was so emotionally stirring that I felt like I'd been hit in the back of the head with a two-by-four. Now you may be surprised to hear a man own up to such an emotional reaction, but let me tell you, we *all* feel like this even though you may not hear many men openly discuss it. From that day forward, I felt like every man, woman, and child on the planet was staring at my hairline. I started noticing people, especially actors on film and TV, and focusing on their hair. Many had toupees that I'd not paid any attention to before, and now I was scrutinizing them and thinking, "My God, you can tell it's a toupee! Is this what I have to look forward to?"

I spent every waking moment aware of my hair loss. No matter what else I was doing, there wasn't a moment when it didn't creep into my thoughts. And at this point my hair loss wasn't even obvious to anyone but me. The sheer anxiety of the idea that my hair loss would progress was, pardon my melodrama, chipping away at my soul.

Like so many others, I began to check out all of the hair loss preventions and remedies I could find. It got to the point where I had an entire file drawer filled with newspaper clippings and ads from magazines. My girlfriend called it my *Paranoid File*. What I didn't realize was that there were millions of other young men suffering in silence just like I was because we've all been forced by society to do so. None of my male friends discussed their hair loss. I figured I was the only man who was bothered about going bald. I figured that the rest of them just "took it like a man" and never let it bother them. How would I know if it bothered them or not? Nobody talked openly about it. Fortunately, this has changed in the dozen or so years since then, in part because I decided to speak up about it and urge others to as well.

Through trial and error and tons of research, I was able to stop the progression of my hair loss and to trigger regrowth. What worked for me was the prescription drug finasteride, first available as Proscar, which is commonly prescribed to treat the prostate, and now available as Propecia, marked specifically for its ability to slow down hair loss and trigger regrowth. I enhanced this treatment with herbal supplements—saw palmetto, *Pygeum africanum*, and stinging nettle—as well as the sugar-balancing (and hormone-balancing) nutritional approach of the diet presented in Dr. Barry Sears' best selling book, *The Zone*.

I began to share my experiences and research with both men and women who were dealing with hair loss and the often unscrupulous hair loss industry. Along the way, I was fortunate to find many dedicated physicians, researchers, and others in the field who are committed to unraveling the mysteries of hair loss and finding successful, healthy treatments. What had begun as a merely personal quest had turned into a full-time job, as I put my broadcast marketing company, Spence-Comm, Inc., on the back burner, and realized I'd become a consumer/patient advocate for the "hair impaired." Now, more than a dozen years after I noticed that first hair fall, I am both optimistic about the future of hair loss research, prevention, and treatments and frustrated by how callously most of the hair loss industry still treats its patients and consumers.

More than fifty million men and twenty million women in the United States alone suffer from "male" pattern baldness and other forms of hair loss. The largely unregulated hair loss industry brings in more than seven billion dollars a year, and unfortunately most of this money is spent on bogus treatments that don't work and transplantation procedures that are harmful, visually unacceptable, and, in many cases, disfiguring. Only a handful of transplant physicians in the country perform state-of-the-art transplants, and you'll find many of them listed at the end of the book in the Resource Guide.

Hair loss is one of the most common, emotionally devastating conditions in the world, and that's because it affects the majority of people on the planet at one time or another in their lives and because those with hair loss are rarely, if ever, taken seriously or treated with any compassion. Men are suffering in silence because they are afraid to admit that their hair loss is a concern to them. Women suffering from hair loss are often even more traumatized than men because they are looked upon by society as abnormal. While a balding man may be extremely disturbed by his appearance, society will not treat him like a freak because he is losing or has lost his hair. We do not stare in shock at a balding man. A woman with thinning hair, however, is met with stares and often feels like an outcast in a society that places an unhealthy, extreme emphasis on a very limited definition of beauty—having a rail-thin body (except for large breasts, of course), flawless features, and luxurious hair.

The Truth About Women's Hair Loss guides you through the often frustrating processes of diagnosis, treatment, and coping with a society and a medical community that are less than supportive of physical and emotional ramifications of hair loss.

Chapter One looks at the many conditions that can cause female hair loss and helps you achieve the proper diagnosis. Chapter Two surveys your treatment options, covering both the pharmaceutical choices and the natural ones. Chapter Three guides you through the hair transplantation procedure and its many controversies, including the reason why so few women make ideal transplantation candidates.

At the end of each of the first three chapters, you'll find important commentary from members of a distinguished panel that includes dedicated, compassionate, and visionary physicians and researchers who are paving the way in diagnosis and treatment. The panel features Dr. Marty Sawaya, one of the country's leading hair loss researchers and hair loss physicians; Dr. Robert M. Bernstein and Dr. William Rassman, who revolutionized hair transplantation with state-of-the-art follicular transplantation; and Dr. Ken Washenik, one of the most respected and knowledgeable physicians specializing in hair loss. Their credentials and contact information are in the Resource Guide.

Chapter Four takes a look at wigs, extensions, and other hair additions that can give you coverage and styling options. Chapter Five looks at the ongoing research into new treatments for women's hair loss. The Appendix provides a list of commonly prescribed drugs that have hair loss as a side effect, looks at the Savin Scale, which measures female hair loss, and includes an exhaustive Resource Guide which provides plenty of practical information and contacts.

I

Why Me? The Causes of Female Hair Loss

You have to accept whatever comes, and the only important thing is that you meet it with courage and with the best you have to give.
—Eleanor Roosevelt

When it comes to female hair loss, the primary issue is that women feel that they are all alone, that no one else is suffering from the condition when, in fact, it is a very common affliction among all women, with more than twenty million affected by various kinds of hair loss in the United States alone. If, for a moment, you put all the other causes aside and just looked at hormonally triggered hair loss, you might be surprised to learn that *the majority of women who have been on birth control pills, who have been pregnant, or who have been through menopause have had to contend with some degree of hair loss.*

Unfortunately, society has forced women to suffer in silence. It is considered far more acceptable for men to go through the same hair loss processes. Even more unfortunately, the medical community also treats the issue of women's hair loss as if it were nonexistent. Since hair loss doesn't appear to be life threatening, most physicians pay little attention to women's complaints about hair loss and essentially tell their patients, "You'll just have to live with it."

Of course, what these physicians don't seem to realize is that the psychological damage caused by hair loss and feeling unattractive can be just as devastating as any serious disease and, in fact, can take an emotional toll that directly affects physical health. Hair loss sufferers experience something truly life altering.

What can you do? If your doctor tells you to "live with it," drop that doctor and do a little research. Find a doctor who will take your situation seriously, someone who is knowledgeable *specifically* about hair loss (most dermatologists have far less training and experience dealing with hair than you might imagine), a dermatologist who devotes most of his or her practice to treating hair loss and other hair problems, someone who will take the time to talk with you and not get you in and out of the office in fifteen minutes and send you home with a bottle of minoxidil without devoting the time to find out the cause of your hair loss and investigate specific treatment options.

You will probably need to find a group of doctors who are willing to work together on your case—a dermatologist, an internist, an endocrinologist (that's a hormone specialist), perhaps your gynecologist, and other specialists as needed. It's very unlikely that one physician will be able to diagnose and treat your condition because *most hair loss is caused by conditions that cross over a few specialties.* In the Resource Guide, you'll find some of the best doctors in the country who are equipped to deal with hair loss in women (see the Hair Loss Physicians section in Appendix C). They can also refer you to doctors in your area.

Diagnosing hair loss properly may take many visits to many kinds of doctors and require second, third, fourth, and even fifth opinions. The process may be frustrating in the beginning. I hope that this book will help guide you.

Understanding Hair

You might think that hair is alive, but it isn't. While hair follicles are alive, hair itself is actually made up of dead cells.

Hair follicles are tiny pockets of live cells just under your skin that are fed by blood vessels that lead into them and by oil glands within the follicles. The oil from these glands also makes your hair shine.

The hair itself is made of a protein called *keratin*, which hardens hair. Keratin also hardens nails, which is why nails can often be affected by certain kinds of hair loss. "Synthesis of proteins requires a great investment of energy," says William R. Rassman, M.D., of our panel of hair loss experts. "When a person becomes ill or malnourished, the hair stops growing; when the illness or malnutrition is severe or prolonged, the hair will even fall out. When hair begins to grow back, that's an early sign that recovery has begun."

Let's take a look at the properties of hair:

• Each strand of hair consists of three layers—the outer *cuticle*, the middle *cortex*, and the inner *medulla*. The cuticle is thin and colorless and protects the thicker cortex, which contains *melanin*, the pigment that colors your hair.

• There are two kinds of melanin. *Eumelanin* makes your hair black or brown, depending upon how much of it your cells pack into each hair. *Pheomelanin* makes your hair red. Blond hair contains very little melanin.

• Melanin is produced by *melanocytes*. When melanocytes can no longer produce as much melanin as is needed to keep the hairs colored because the *tyrosinase* enzymes that create melanin are lost, hair will turn white. Stress and physical illness can accelerate the graying process.

• Human hair is classified into two main types. *Vellus* hair is fine and can range from "peach fuzz" to hairs that are so fine they're almost invisible except upon very close or microscopic inspection. *Terminal* hair is the coarser, longer, more visible hair. Except for the palms of the hands and the soles of the feet, most of the human body is covered with hair.

• The shape of the cortex in cross section determines whether hair will be straight, wavy, or curly. A cylindrical cross section is found in straight hair, an oval one in curly hair. Slight variations in these cross section shapes determine degrees of straightness, waviness, and curliness.

• The inner medulla reflects light, giving hair its color tones.

• Most of your hair's qualities are controlled by heredity.

• The average head has one hundred thousand hair follicles, but they are not all in the same growth phase at the same time. Hair grows about half an inch each month. Each strand will grow at this pace for about two to seven years in what is called the *anagen* phase. Then each strand rests for a while in the *catagen* phase. It falls out in the *telogen* phase, which is often referred to as the *shedding phase*. Don't be confused if you hear *telogen* referred to as a *resting phase*. In that instance, *telogen* applies to the hair *follicle*, which is resting when a hair sheds. When a strand falls out, another one is right behind it, about to break the surface of your scalp. At any given time, 90 percent of your hairs are in the growing phase.

• Normal hair loss in this cycle is between fifty and one hundred strands per day.

• Hair falls out and is replaced at staggered intervals from follicles all over your head, so that natural, cyclical hair loss is never noticed. You won't lose just front, top, side, or back hair at the end of a cycle—hair falls out at various times from all parts of your head.

• Hormones' effects are not limited to causing hair loss or preventing it. Higher levels of hormones can mean higher levels of oil in your hair follicles' oil glands. Hormonal changes during pregnancy can cause hair to become more oily and can change curly hair to straight hair. Sometimes this change in curliness is permanent.

Varieties of Women's Hair Loss

Hair loss can be temporary or long lasting. Temporary hair loss can be easy to fix when its cause is identified and dealt with or difficult when it is not immediately clear what the cause is. Hair loss that could have been merely temporary may become long lasting as a result of an incorrect diagnosis. The potential for such misdiagnoses is perhaps the most frustrating aspect of hair loss for women. The information in this chapter will help you identify the cause of your hair loss and ideally lead you and your doctors to the right treatments for your particular kind of hair loss sooner rather than later.

Alopecia is the medical term for excessive or abnormal hair loss. There are different kinds of alopecia. What all hair loss has in common, whether it's in men or women, is that *it is always a symptom of something else that's gone wrong in your body*. Your hair will remain on your head where it belongs if hormone imbalance, disease, or some other condition is not occurring. That condition may be as simple as having a gene that makes you susceptible to male or female pattern baldness or one of the forms of alopecia areata. Or it may be as complex as a whole host of diseases. Fortunately, hair loss may also be a symptom of a short-term event such as stress, pregnancy, and the taking of certain medications. In these situations, hair will grow back when the event has passed. Substances (including hormones), medications, and diseases can cause a change in the hair growth and shedding phases and in their durations. When this happens, synchronous growth and shedding occur. Once the cause is dealt with, hairs go back to their random pattern of growth and shedding, and your hair loss problem stops.

Causes of Hair Loss

Let's take a look at the causes of hair loss.

The Hormone Connection

Dihydrotestosterone (DHT), a derivative of the male hormone testosterone, is the enemy of hair follicles on your head. Simply put, under certain conditions DHT wants those follicles dead. This simple action is at the root (pardon the pun) of many kinds of hair loss, so we'll address it first.

Androgenetic alopecia, commonly called *male* or *female pattern baldness*, was only partially understood until the last few decades. For many years, scientists thought that androgenetic alopecia was caused by the predominance of the male sex hormone, testosterone, which women also have in trace amounts under normal conditions. While testosterone is at the core of the balding process, DHT is thought to be the main culprit.

Testosterone converts to DHT with the aid of the enzyme Type II 5-alpha reductase, which is held in a hair follicle's oil glands. Scientists now believe that it's not the amount of circulating testosterone that's the problem but the level of DHT binding to receptors in scalp follicles. DHT shrinks hair follicles, making it impossible for healthy hair to survive.

There are natural and herbal treatments and now drugs on the market that can curb hair loss and prompt regrowth because of their ability to interfere with DHT's follicle-killing mission by either inhibiting 5-alpha reductase, and therefore the amount of DHT that can be created out of testosterone, or by inhibiting DHT's ability to bind to receptors in hair follicles. DHT is also the main culprit in prostate problems, which is why many natural treatments and drugs that are used to treat the prostate might also be used to prevent or treat hair loss.

The hormonal process of testosterone converting to DHT, which then harms hair follicles, happens in both men and women. Under normal conditions, women have a minute fraction of the level of testosterone that men have, but even a lower level can cause DHT-triggered hair loss in women. And certainly when those levels rise, DHT is even more of a problem. Those levels can rise and still be within what doctors consider "normal" on a blood test, even though they are high enough to cause a problem. The levels may not rise at all and still be a problem if you have the kind of body chemistry that is overly sensitive to even its regular levels of chemicals, including hormones.

Since hormones operate in the healthiest manner when they are in a delicate balance, the *androgens*, as male hormones are called, do not need to be raised to trigger a problem. Their counterpart female hormones, when lowered, give an edge to these androgens, such as DHT. Such an imbalance can also cause problems, including hair loss.

Interestingly, DHT behaves differently at various sites on the body. The pattern baldness areas of the head—the front, temples, and crown—are more sensitive to testosterone and therefore quicker to convert it to DHT. As DHT shrinks a hair follicle, shortening a hair's growth cycle, a normal hair's diameter lessens and lessens over time until the hair is tiny and fine. Ultimately, no hair can grow when the follicle goes completely dormant or dies. DHT behaves quite differently elsewhere on the body. It's actually thought to stimulate hair growth in follicles on the chest, back, shoulders, eyebrows, and ears.

Geographical and cultural influences also affect hormones. Compared to Asian men, for example, Americans have more 5-alpha reductase, the enzyme that converts testosterone to DHT, and therefore have more body hair and more baldness. Scientists are studying the link that a culture's food choices may play in the action of our hormones—a diet higher in fat that does not keep blood sugar constantly balanced may create conditions in the follicles' oil glands that lead to the production of more 5-alpha reductase.

Baldness can also be self-perpetuating. In balding areas, the oil glands in the hair follicle become larger. Since these glands also hold the enzyme that converts testosterone to DHT, there's always a lot of the enzyme in these enlarged glands in balding areas, poised to further weaken the hair follicles. Oil gland activity is also increased by higher amounts of circulating hormones.

Hormones are cyclical. Testosterone levels in some men drop by 10 percent each decade after thirty. Women's hormone levels decline as menopause approaches and drop sharply during menopause and beyond.

Testosterone levels peak in the fall and are lowest in the spring. During the spring low, hair grows the most. As testosterone levels rise, heading toward fall, so does hair loss. By fall, twice as much hair is lost than was lost in the spring. Both men and women have a similar hair growth seasonal cycle. The cyclic nature of both our hair and hormones is one reason hair loss can increase in the short term even when you are experiencing a long-term slowdown of hair loss (and a long-term increase in hair growth) while on a treatment that controls hair loss.

Diffuse Alopecia

Telogen Effluvium
When your body goes through something traumatic, like childbirth, malnutrition, a severe infection, major surgery, or extreme

stress, many of the 90 percent of your hairs that are currently in the growing (*anagen*) phase or catagen (resting) phase can shift all at once to the shedding (*telogen*) phase. About three months after the event that triggered this shift, many of those 90 percent fall out at the same time. This phenomenon is called *telogen effluvium*. No treatment is usually needed since the hairs will all immediately begin the growing phase again. Some women, however, have chronic telogen effluvium, and treatments must be based upon what caused the "trauma" in the first place and upon the persistent conditions that may be contributing to this kind of continuous shedding.

Anagen Effluvium

This is the hair loss associated with chemotherapy. Since chemotherapy targets your body's rapidly dividing cancer cells, your body's other rapidly dividing cells, such as hair follicles in the growing (anagen) phase, are also greatly affected. Soon after chemotherapy begins, 90 percent or more of the hairs can fall out while still in the anagen phase.

Androgenetic Alopecia (Female Pattern Baldness)

The majority of women with androgenetic alopecia have diffuse thinning on all areas of the head. Men, on the other hand, rarely have diffuse thinning but instead have thinning in the front, top, and crown areas. Some women may have a combination of the two pattern types. Androgenetic alopecia in women is due to the action of androgens, male hormones that are typically present in only small amounts (see The Hormone Connection on page 6). Androgenetic alopecia can be caused by a variety of factors tied to the actions of hormones, including an androgen-secreting tumor, ovarian cysts, the taking of high androgen index birth controls pills, pregnancy, menopause, hormone imbalance (including one caused by the thyroid), and even the body's over-reaction to "normal" hormone levels. Some women with androgenetic alopecia, especially those who have androgen-secreting tumors or ovarian cysts, may also have other androgenetic symptoms besides hair loss. These include acne, excess facial and body hair, and menstrual irregularities.

Patchy Alopecia (Alopecia Areata)

There are three kinds of patchy alopecia: *alopecia areata* (the most common of the three) in which patches of scalp hair fall out; *alopecia totalis* in which all scalp hair is lost; and *alopecia universalis* in which all scalp and body hair are lost.

At any one time, 0.05 percent to 0.10 percent of the population is affected by alopecia areata. That's between 112,000 and 224,000 people in the United States and between 2.25 and 4.50 million worldwide.

The exact cause of alopecia areata is not known, and it may take years for the condition to be fully understood. Currently, the prevailing theory is that it may be an autoimmune disorder, meaning that the immune system attacks something in the body as if it were a foreign invader—in this case, hair follicles. The evidence for areata as an immune disease is entirely circumstantial: The fact that there is an immune system response at the hair follicles may suggest an immune disorder, yet scientists admit that this evidence comes nowhere near to proving the theory. If it's not an immune disorder, what might cause alopecia areata? The immune system may actually have a good reason to attack the follicles, one that just hasn't been identified yet. For example, perhaps in the follicles there is a virus or some other culprit.

One of the clues that this may *not* be an autoimmune disease is that the attacked tissue, the hair follicle, is *not* destroyed; it just stops producing hair above the scalp. The follicles still produce root material and often even hair, but it's too small and abnormal to work its way above the skin. In someone with alopecia areata, the hair follicles are said to be in a state called *dystrophic anagen*.

Alopecia areata may also be genetic. In 20 percent of the cases, there is a family history of the condition. It may also be linked to stress.

Alopecia areata affects men and women equally at all ages, including childhood, and can occur gradually, first showing up as broken hairs that taper to a thinner end, or quickly, with a small, completely bald patch showing up within twenty-four hours.

There is no conclusive diagnostic test, and doctors typically rule out other causes and kinds of hair loss before diagnosing alopecia areata or alopecia totalis and universalis, which are progressions of alopecia areata. However, some people feel a tingling sensation or pain in conjunction with alopecia areata. Others feel nothing.

Alopecia areata research has been slow, and only in the last fifteen years have major attempts been made to understand and define it. Much of the interest has been sparked by the efforts of the National Alopecia Areata Foundation. Still, only about twenty research groups worldwide are currently focusing on the condition, and there is little money available for research. Some of the current research is aimed at the genetics of alopecia areata and at developing new treatments.

Trichotillomania

Trichotillomania is the condition of twisting and pulling out one's own hair. This behavior is usually seen in children or adolescents; it is found in adults less frequently. It's associated with psychological stress or disorder. Some affected people don't even consciously realize that they're pulling out their hair. Several years of this behavior destroys the hair follicles so that they can't grow hair properly at all. Psychologically based treatments are usually suggested.

Traction Alopecia

This condition is caused by localized trauma to the hair follicles from tight hairstyles that pull at hair over time. If the condition is detected early enough, the hair will regrow. Braiding, corn-rows, tight ponytails, and extensions are the most common styling causes.

Patchy Alopecia with Scarring

Unlike alopecia areata, this patchy alopecia occurs with scarring on the scalp. It can be congenital (present at birth); result from trauma, including burns, frostbite, injury, and radiation; or result from infection or inflammation. It may be associated with the pressure sores suffered by someone bedridden and unconscious or simply have no known cause.

Congenital Triangular Alopecia

This condition is often confused with alopecia areata. Congen-ital triangular alopecia is a patch of hair loss in the temple area. It is found mainly in children any time from birth to about five years. It's nonprogressive, noninflammatory, and nonscarring.

Loose Hair Syndrome

Also known as *loose anagen syndrome* or *loose anagen hair*, this condition is noninflammatory and nonscarring, and it most often affects children. It can be patchy or diffuse, and when it's exten-sive, it affects the back of the scalp far more than the front. This may be from the back of the head rubbing against a pillow.

In this syndrome, hair is loose and easily pulls out of the follicles. The remaining hair doesn't grow very long and can be unruly and hard to comb or style. This condition most often affects blond hair.

The affected hairs are still in the active growth phase, but their root sheaths, which normally surround and protect the hair shafts, aren't produced properly in the follicles, so hair is poorly anchored. First identified in 1986, this condition can be genetic and run in families. It can improve on its own as an affected child ages, but if the condition doesn't develop until the child is five years old or older, the hair loss will be more persistent.

Inflammatory Alopecias

Pseudopelade
Also known as *alopecia cicatrisata*, this is a rare condition that primarily affects women and sometimes children. Pseudopelade is an inflammation of the upper portion of the hair follicle, while alopecia areata's inflammation occurs primarily around the lower part of the hair follicle. While alopecia areata can progress indefinitely, pseudopelade causes hair loss over several years and then stops, resulting in bald patches where the follicles have been damaged. Once the progression of hair loss stops, so does the inflammation in the upper portion of the hair follicle.

Scleroderma
An autoimmune disease, scleroderma is a gradual hardening and tightening of the skin that can also cause hair loss. As it progresses, the hardening can spread throughout the body to affect joints, muscles, and organs.

Tick Bites
When hair loss occurs in the area of a tick bite, it is temporary. The hair will regrow when the inflammation subsides.

Lichen Planus

Most often seen in middle-aged adults, this condition produces pink papules on the skin and scalp. These papules have a shiny, smooth, flat surface and can expand to form pink, violet, or brown plaques. The hair inside these plaques can be lost. Lichen planus can be confused with hair loss from systematic lupus in skin biopsies, so great care must be taken in making a diagnosis.

Psoriasis

Hair loss caused by psoriasis can occur when the affected patches of skin have hair follicles that have been forced into the hair shedding phase.

Lupus

Systemic lupus erythematosus (SLE) is a rare, chronic disease in which many organ systems—including the skin, joints, heart, lungs, kidneys, brain, and blood vessels—become inflamed. It is an autoimmune disorder whose cause is unknown. Women are affected far more than men in a ratio of ten to one. Diffuse hair loss may occur and may change according to the severity of the disease. In some cases, the hair loss may be permanent.

Seborrheic Dermatitis

This is an inflammation of the skin caused when the oil glands attached to the hair follicles begin to produce excessive amounts of sebum (oil). Triggered by hormone fluctuation, this kind of dermatitis can also cause temporary hair loss.

Iron Overload (Hemochromatosis)

Iron overload can be caused by a high intake of iron or by the genetic disease hemochromatosis, in which the body isn't able to break down and remove iron from the bloodstream. Hair loss can be a symptom of this serious disease. Hemochromatosis can be treated once diagnosed but can be life threatening when undiagnosed. All people who experience the onset of hair loss should ask their doctors to check their iron levels as a precaution.

Hair Loss from Cancer

Chemotherapy used to treat cancer may result in hair loss, but so can some cancers themselves, including skin cancers that destroy hair follicles or spread to them and cancers that originate elsewhere but spread to the skin and destroy the hair follicles. Cancers can disrupt the normal hormone activity and balance, causing hair loss. Cancer also depletes the body's resources, vitamins, minerals, and energy, leading to the loss of hair in a gradual, diffuse manner (see Telogen Effluvium). These kinds of hair loss do not involve permanent damage to hair follicles, and the hair usually returns after the cancer is successfully treated.

Diagnostic Tests

When a doctor performs tests to diagnose hair loss, he or she should test the following:

• hormone levels (DHEAs, testosterone, androstenedione, prolactin, follicular stimulating hormone, and leutinizing hormone)

• serum iron

• serum ferritin

• total iron binding capacity (TIBC)

• thyroid stimulating hormone (T3, T4, TSH)

• VDRL

• complete blood count (CBC)

- scalp biopsy

- hair pull

- densitometry (to check for miniaturization of the hair shaft under extreme magnification)

Panel Commentary on Diagnosing Hair Loss

Dr. Marty Sawaya

- "Women can have lots of different hair problems; women don't all suffer from the same problem. I see women who've had hair loss from hair processing, including chemical treatments, coloring, and perms. Then there's that group of women who have chronic shedding problems from other causes. And there's the group who have female pattern hair loss, just as men have male pattern hair loss. There's also a smaller group of women who have scarring on their scalps from years of chemical processing. Not all dermatologists recognize the causes of women's hair loss, and they just throw them into one category and that's why the patients get such jumbled up treatment. Of course, it would be so much easier if the women found the right doctor to treat them from the very beginning. So women have a rougher time with diagnosing and treating hair loss because it's not like men's hair loss where 80 percent to 90 percent have the same cause—androgenetic alopecia, also called *pattern baldness*, in this case *male*."

- "Stress is a contributing factor when you have a hair loss problem. Stress changes the immune system and that adversely affects the hair follicle."

- "Doctors need to spend at least an hour with each patient when working on a diagnosis. Unfortunately, doctors don't or can't take that kind of time anymore—they get their patients in and out in five minutes—and they don't take the time to talk about what may be causing the problem and how to approach treatment. Remember, each patient is unique. I had a patient the other day who had just seen a colleague of mine, one who is one of the experts at a major university, and the doctor just walked in and told the patient, 'This is what you have,' and then was out of there in five minutes. She didn't spend any time with the patient and talk to her. And the patient *didn't* have the condition the doctor thought she had. This is very frustrating. There's not one diagnosis, one straight kitchen book formula, for everybody."

• "If you are getting a biopsy it certainly is not helpful if a general pathologist reads it. The biopsy has to be specially done to gain some insight into your particular scalp problem. The traditional way is to cut the biopsies vertically, but now we're recognizing that horizontally is a much better approach. The general pathologist or derm pathologist can't read it though. It has to be specially read by one of the few in the country who know how to do that."

• "Patients face a big problem when they go to a general practitioner or dermatologist who isn't adequately trained in hair. High androgen/male hormone index birth control pills can start the ball rolling on hair loss, yet the average gynecologist who prescribes this is not in tune to the hair effects caused by oral contraceptives because their only concern is from the waist down!"

• "One of the biggest problems with diagnosing female pattern hair loss—androgenetic alopecia—is that it overlaps tremendously with chronic telogen effluvium." [Both conditions are described earlier in this chapter.]

• "There is so much misinformation out there, and a patient's ability to get to the *right* sources is the main problem."

Dr. Ken Washenik

• "When I meet with a patient, I really have to listen to her history, find out if her hair loss has been acute in its onset or slow and gradual over the years, see if it's associated with any other scalp problems, like itching, pain, dandruff, or scaling. I ask what her treatment history has been, then take a history of her hormonal background, her menstrual cycles too. The main concern is *Where is this going to lead? Am I going bald?* That's followed by *Why is this happening? It hasn't happened before. Why is it happening now?* When patients come in they are justifiably afraid. They have some shedding hair or they have enough thinness that they can see some scalp and they're concerned that they are going to go completely bald. Fortunately, it's rare for a woman with androgenetic alopecia to go bald like a man goes bald. But first you have to determine if it's androgenetic alopecia or another kind. This gives you a sense of whether they can get their hair back."

• "I just can't describe how catastrophic hair loss is to my female patients."

Dr. William Rassman

• "Many doctors don't recognize a woman's hair loss even when it's there to see. Most women end up going from doctor to doctor and even get sent to psychiatrists."

• "More women than men are prone to what I call *fragile hair syndrome*. It's not unusual to find that these women lose hair during periods of stress because stress impairs the immune system. They can lose significant amounts of hair, but it's temporary and once the stress or crisis passes, the hair will grow back."

2

What Can I Do? Treatments for Women's Hair Loss

To become successful you must become a person of action. Merely to know is not sufficient. It is necessary both to know and to do.
—Napoleon Hill

The practice of medicine is sexist. That shouldn't surprise you, since everything else in our society is too. But while the drug companies aren't working specifically on women's hair loss, there is hope.

Keep in mind that medicine is an industry, that drug companies are *businesses*, and that economics is behind each and every decision made by them regarding treatments for any condition, including hair loss. Men are foremost on everyone's mind in commerce, no matter what the products and services. When it comes to hair loss, that is the rule too, and it is most unfortunate.

There is not one drug designed specifically for hair loss in women. Some of the drugs designed for men *will* help women though, and in some cases even more than they do men! Minoxidil, the topical lotion sold under the brand name Rogaine, is a good example of that interesting phenomenon. By the time you read this, an extra-strength Rogaine specifically tested on and marketed to women will be available. It is the exact same drug as the one for men, but because of FDA drug testing regulations, it had to be thoroughly tested on women before it could be approved for sale to them because it had first been developed solely as a man's hair loss treatment. Minoxidil didn't start its life as a hair loss drug. It was used to treat high blood pressure. Hair growth was reported as a side effect, so its use as a hair loss treatment was then researched and tested.

None of the new hair loss drugs currently in the testing phase in the United States are designed specifically for women and their particular physiology. In Europe this isn't the case— their scientists *are* designing and testing hair loss drugs specifically for women, and ideally some of those will make their way through the politics and the bureaucracy to become available in the United States one day.

Many natural treatments are more effective and safer than pharmaceutical drugs, although for economic reasons until very recently the pharmaceutical industry was doing everything it could to discredit anything used medicinally unless it was a pharmaceutical. That situation is slowly changing, again for economic reasons.

"More than 25 percent of our mainstream pharmaceuticals are derived from plants, and 60 percent have additional plant-based ingredients," reports journalist and author Nina L. Diamond in her book *Purify Your Body: Natural Remedies for Detoxing from 50 Everyday Situations.* "We already know the chemical properties of many other herbs and botanicals that heal or positively affect the body and mind. These are used in natural treatments but aren't yet being synthesized into pharmaceuticals."

If herbs, botanicals, and other natural substances are medicinally active and actually work, why do drug companies bother to create synthetic versions of them, adding other chemicals in the process (which often produce side effects the natural versions wouldn't have had) and sometimes even weakening the healing abilities of the natural substance, and turn them into prescription or over-the-counter drugs?

Money, money, money. You can't claim ownership of a plant, botanical, or nutrient and then patent it. So, for purely economic reasons, drug companies synthesize many of these natural substances and create a brand-new human-made compound, which they can then claim exclusive ownership of by obtaining a patent. That patent gives them the right to be the only company that can sell the drug for a number of years (can you hear the cash registers ringing?) until the patent expires, at which point other drug companies can also manufacture and sell the drug.

Faced with an explosion of competition from herbs, botanicals, and nutrients in their natural form, as their active medicinal properties are scientifically documented and more people are incorporating them into all areas of their health care, the pharmaceutical companies finally woke up to the old adage "If you can't beat 'em, join 'em." So, many pharmaceutical companies now have divisions that sell natural, herbal products, the very same products that they were trying to discredit just a couple of years ago. None of these products can be owned exclusively by any one company, so many brands are available, not only from these new divisions of drug companies, but also from the many companies that have dominated the natural treatment market for years—those companies that don't manufacture and market pharmaceuticals but only make herbal, botanical, and other natural products such as vitamins, minerals, and nutritional supplements.

"At least twenty thousand scientific papers have been published in journals that attest to the efficacy" of herbal, botanical, and nutritional treatment regarding health, Diamond notes in *Purify Your Body*. "In Europe, particularly Germany, scientists, medical researchers, physicians, and health practitioners are way, way ahead of the United States in this area."

The United States has been "officially" trying to catch up since creating the Office of Alternative Medicine (OAM) at the National Institutes of Health (NIH) in 1992. The OAM funds research and clinical studies of a wide array of natural treatments, although its funding budget is minuscule compared to the budgets of other areas of the NIH.

Actually, what has been labeled alternative medicine is our *original* medicine. Natural treatments were our *only* medicine until just about one hundred years ago when the modern pharmaceutical company system of creating medicines came into being. Of course, we wouldn't want to be without many of these synthesized pharmaceutical drugs that can be truly life saving, but natural treatments should not be excluded since they can be better suited to our medicinal needs and often have a vastly lowered risk of side effects. Keep in mind, though, that herbs, botanicals, nutrients, and other natural treatments are powerful. After all, that's why they work. So they should be used as carefully as any other kind of "drug."

Women have far fewer pharmaceutical options than men for dealing with hair loss. For this reason, women more often call upon natural treatments when trying to prevent or treat hair loss and its causes.

Women's Experiences with Diagnosis and Treatment

You are not alone in your quest to find the proper diagnosis and treatment for your hair loss. The medical community is finally under enough pressure to take hair loss and, more specifically, women's hair loss more seriously and to provide a better informed standard of care. Millions of women are sharing their stories and frustrations with each other. Even more importantly, they are speaking publicly about the need for more research, more physicians specializing in hair loss, more treatment options, and more of *everything* that other medical specialties can offer their patients but that hair loss as a specialty has been sadly lacking.

"For a problem that is so devastating, female hair loss has received very little attention from the medical community," wrote men's hair loss pioneer O'Tar Norwood, M.D., in a recent letter to me. Norwood, the creator of the Norwood Scale, the standard by which men's hair loss is measured, added, "Little is known about its etiology and treatment. Maybe your book will stimulate interest to help these women."

Dr. Norwood and I have had many discussions about hair loss in the past few years, and he is among those in the medical community calling for increased attention to the causes and treatments of women's hair loss.

Every day I hear from men and women around the world regarding their hair loss. They call my office, they write, they call my radio program, and they E-mail me. I receive nearly one thousand E-mails every week. In this section I will share with you some of the experiences of the women who have E-mailed me recently. I hope that hearing about these women's experiences will help you in your efforts to prevent and treat hair loss. You may see some of your own experiences in the stories these women share.

Here are the common elements that haunt so many women trying to get the proper diagnosis and treatment:

• virtually useless blood tests that have such a broad "normal" range that they rarely help in diagnosis

• a system in which labs are *not* standardized, so two labs may send back very different results for the exact same blood sample

• the lack of knowledge on the part of doctors about hair loss, its causes, and more accurate testing methods, including the saliva test that measures hormone levels often far more accurately than does a blood test and without having that deceivingly wide so-called "normal" range

• the lack of understanding that even though a patient may fall into a "normal" category doesn't mean that her levels aren't causing a problem in her system

• the lack of caring by many doctors, some of whom are trained so well to maintain a professional distance that they are in fact cold and callous

• many doctors' attitudes that they can cover up their ignorance about hair loss and its causes and treatments by claiming, "There's nothing wrong with you," rather than admit that they have not been taught much about this area

• the refusal of doctors, even dermatologists who are supposed to know the most about hair, to take hair loss seriously

It is my sincere hope that in the near future medical schools will expand their dermatology coursework, clinical teachings, and residency programs to include areas that will make them truly qualified to understand and treat hair loss. Doctors must have better education in the body's systems that trigger hair loss. Many dermatologists are themselves frustrated by their lack of training in this area.

Stress is the common catchall diagnosis when a doctor doesn't feel equipped to really study a patient's health and the causes of her hair loss. How many women have spent five minutes with a doctor who simply looked at them and said, "It's probably just stress," and then sent them on their merry way? Millions upon millions. It is appalling that so many doctors encourage their patients to medicate their *concern* about hair loss by recommending antidepressant drugs rather than taking the hair loss problem seriously and trying to diagnose its cause and determine its proper treatment. The greatest irony is that most of the commonly prescribed antidepressants have hair loss as a *major* side effect!

Rarely is hair loss due *just* to stress. While stress can trigger a temporary bout with hair loss, it is absolutely imperative that doctors spend as much time as it takes to thoroughly investigate all of the systemic possible causes of a woman's hair loss.

The women who share their stories here speak in their own words for millions just like them.

Kathleen's Story

Kathleen runs one of the women's hair loss support groups on the Internet.

Hair loss can many times be a gift, because if you can tackle the issue of hair loss and get better health because of it, you will benefit. You will also learn compassion, and how not to judge people from the outside. It's going to prepare you for greater issues that you may have to face in your life. You'll walk through those, too, and you'll survive them as well.

Find a support system, find other women who are also facing hair loss. Often when we only talk about this to our friends and family who are not experiencing hair loss they get tired of hearing about it.

Testing can be very frustrating. Blood tests rarely reveal anything because their so-called "normal" range is too broad and misses most problems causing hair loss. Saliva tests can be more accurate. You'll need to be tested not only for hormone levels but down to mineral levels as well.

Lucy's Story

I'm forty-three and in past years I've had a few episodes of telogen effluvium—usually three-month episodes of sudden shedding, followed by regrowth. I've had six such episodes between the ages of nineteen and forty, but now it's been shedding for eleven months. I assumed this was another episode of telogen effluvium, but it hasn't passed. It never lasted this long in the past and I never lost this much hair. I had the flu, and a high fever of 103, a month prior to the beginning of this shedding. While most of the physicians I've seen think that chronic telogen effluvium is the cause, some physicians feel that there may be an additional problem, perhaps androgenetic alopecia (male/female pattern baldness). All of my blood tests have come back "normal." I don't have polycystic ovaries, adrenal hyperplasia, lupus, or any of the scarring alopecias.

My fear and uncertainty are overwhelming.

In addition to having trouble obtaining a definitive diagnosis, I've found that each doctor has an entirely different idea regarding treatment, which causes considerable confusion. Every doctor prescribes something else and contradicts what another doctor has prescribed. Each physician can look at my scalp—even on the same day—and diagnose something else! Each doctor is into his or her own protocol and feels that his or her method, regime, or products are the only ones that work. And then there are those physicians who are not very optimistic about female hair loss altogether.

Aren't there any guidelines in this field?

I want to be able to help myself, but I do not even know what is causing this. I have had many negative reactions to many medications and have had prescription drugs trigger hair loss in the past. I would feel a lot better if I knew what was truly going on so I could target treatment more appropriately before taking a systemic medication, which could make things worse. I always took exceptionally good care of my hair. I've even had my thick hair waist length. So you can't begin to imagine how I feel now. A couple of months ago someone commented that I had long, beautiful hair. I hadn't heard that in a while, and I thanked the person and then burst out crying. I cried for two hours because I knew that I probably would never have nice hair again. Just recently a doctor who had no compassion told me to chop all my hair off above my ears "like a man," he said. I felt sick—he had absolutely no understanding. His assistant told me not to step back into their office unless I had cut off all my hair. She was so cruel, and I felt so vulnerable. I knew it wasn't necessary to cut off all my hair. It reminded me of the first time I had telogen effluvium and ran to a doctor with a bag of hair. He looked at my full head of thick hair and accused me of lying and told me I should be ashamed of myself. I cried. This rips you apart and destroys any sense of security. In my mind, I know hair is not a vital body part like an arm, a leg, or a breast, but my heart doesn't know the difference and I feel such pain. Although others probably can't tell at this point, I am still very self-conscious especially in bright sunlight and certain indoor lighting.

My husband and family say that they can't tell, but they may be just telling me that. With this much hair falling out, I feel as though it is only a matter of time.

This destroys your sense of self, your self-esteem, your confidence, and sense of femininity. And it robs you of your dignity when you have to deal with these doctors. It stresses a marriage and your family. There is very little emotional support for women with hair loss. We live in a society that relates to women based on appearance, and that makes this so difficult. If you lose a vital organ or part of your body, you are allowed to grieve, but society deems it unacceptable to grieve for your hair.

Tammy's Story

I'm in good shape, thirty-nine, and have no other physical problems. No heredity hair loss in my family either. That's why I'm at such a loss. I'm losing my hair and I've gotten nowhere with doctors. I've been going to a so-called "expert" for almost a year who still can't give me a diagnosis. If I ask questions, this doctor gets indignant and is on a major ego trip. I really don't know what to do.

Susan's Story

Almost a year ago, I first realized that I was losing my hair. I don't ever remember feeling so frightened in all my life. For days, I just couldn't pull myself together. I couldn't stop crying. I didn't dare comb, wash, or even touch my hair. When my appointment with my doctor came around, I sat shaking in the chair and blurted out that I thought I was going bald. I began to cry. He offered me a tissue and some reassurance, then looked at my hair and scalp with some kind of lens and told me not to worry. Not to worry?

Who wouldn't worry when their hair is coming out in handfuls? He ordered some blood tests and said I was suffering from stress. He told me to come back in two weeks for the blood test results.

Those two weeks seemed like forever. I just wanted to know what the tests showed. I wanted to know that I could be treated for whatever was causing my hair to fall out. I wanted to stop my hair from falling out.

I didn't know back then how naïve and trusting I was.

The two weeks finally passed and I was back in the chair. "All your blood tests are normal. You're a little low on iron, so we will treat that, but besides that you're fine," said my doctor.

Fine? How could I be fine? My hair was coming out at an alarming rate. Surely I would be bald by Christmas. How could I possibly be fine?

I walked out of the doctor's office with a prescription for an iron supplement and a diagnosis of stress.

The weeks went by and my hair was as bad as ever. Now I was very concerned. I decided to see another doctor, this time a female physician. She just held up her hands and said she would refer me to a dermatologist at the local hospital. I had to wait a month before my appointment. By now I was beginning to get a sinking feeling that I wasn't going to get much help here. I didn't feel that I was being taken seriously. My doctor was making me feel about ten years old with his attitude. I had to do more to help myself, so I decided to try to find out what was going on. I never did believe it was stress that was causing my hair to fall out. This was something more than that. And so began my round of visits to all the local libraries, libraries in every town or city I visited, bookstores in and out of town. I spent hours searching the Internet for information and visited hundreds of sites.

I also talked to people. I wanted to know everything I could, so I had to ask questions. I was open about what I was going through, and I soon realized I wasn't the only woman to experience hair loss. It was around this time that I found the AOL (America Online) support group/board. I was shocked, to say the least. So many women experiencing the same as me, all with a similar story to tell.

How could this be? Why wasn't there more help and answers from the doctors for all these women? I just couldn't take it all in. And here I was at the other side of the country and even the world from all of these women, and we're all in the same position—we're not being taken seriously or being heard. This was not right. At least I was no longer alone in this.

My first appointment with the dermatologist wasn't exactly what I was expecting. In fact, I think I came out of there in a state of shock. Without even getting out of his chair, the dermatologist told me that I would probably never get my hair back, and that he would refer me to a psychiatrist who would give me some antidepressants. What the hell was going on here? I needed help with my hair loss, not my mind. I felt so insulted. He didn't even know me. He said he could do another blood test and see me in a month. I just walked out. I knew by now that I was not the only woman having these dreadful experiences with doctors who knew nothing about hair loss.

The second blood test showed again that everything was in that broad "normal" range. Well, I sure as hell didn't think everything was so normal. Everything I suggested to my dermatologist was just brushed aside, and he said, "I think it's just stress."

These visits to my dermatologist were just a joke, and it makes me ill to think that these people can treat their patients with such contempt. This doctor belittled me with callous humor. "Well, you look lovely to me. You're fine," the doctor said, laughing from behind the desk.

I live in England and had come to the end of the line with our health care system. Now what? I knew that I was on my own. It was up to me.

During all of this, I never stopped looking and trying to learn and understand what could be going on. I had narrowed down the conditions that could be causing my hair loss to just two. I felt that I was at least getting somewhere.

I had read so much by now and learned a lot that made sense to me. I had always felt that my hair loss could be related to a hormone imbalance, since I had some other symptoms as well. After reading about a particular saliva hormone test, I thought that it should be my next move. The test wasn't available in England. I spoke to my doctor about it, but his response was the same as it had always been: very negative and condescending. He wanted nothing to do with the tests and refused to even look at the results once I had them.

I went ahead with the tests, which I had performed via a U.S. lab. Now I needed a doctor who would look at the results of the tests, work with me, and hopefully find an end to my problem.

I had come across a few names on the Internet and made a note of them. Again, it felt good to know that even women in the United States were going through the same frustrations as I was, as we shared our experiences on the on-line support group. I spent a day in a city library and found the names of a few other doctors. I went to my favorite bookstore and found a book with another listing of doctors, and one of them — Dr. Shirley Bond — was the same as one from my Internet list. I researched her and found out that she is a highly qualified and insightful doctor. She was well known, in particular, for women's health and for her knowledge about the role of the hormone progresterone in women's health, which is largely ignored by doctors in both the United States and in England. The hormone test that I had had was a saliva test, known to be even more accurate in many instances than those blood tests with their very broad so-called "normal ranges."

I made an appointment to see her in London. She was just as I had imagined, as wonderful as everything I had read about her. I took with me all the copies of the blood tests I had done and the results of the saliva test, which she would be the first to read. My saliva tests showed that I was very low in progesterone. After a half-hour consultation with Dr. Bond, she decided to put me on natural progesterone, initially for two months, and then we would see how I do.

That is where I am today. After a frustrating and often lonely year, after discovering the appalling manner in which women can often be treated by the medical profession, I have finally found a doctor who will listen to me and respect me and who is on my side.

Janet's Story

I'm twenty-six years old and have been suffering from hair loss since I was in the eighth grade. I can't believe how people think that women's hair loss isn't compelling and important — that really burns me up. There are so many more women out there dealing with this devastating problem than people realize. It has always been such a man's issue and has only been given attention when hair loss applies to men. As a woman dealing with this, I have virtually nowhere to go for help, and neither do so many other women. We're all on our own, finding each other in support groups and on the Internet, swapping stories about treatments that work and those that don't, about possible causes. We end up far more concerned and knowledgeable than the professionals, the doctors! Personally, I feel like a freak of nature sometimes—a woman losing her hair, and at this young an age. Come on. It's not normal. I find myself thinking about this a lot, especially when I see women with beautiful hair and I envy it so much.

Everyone in my family has a full head of hair. None of them have this problem but me. I ask myself why, but I do not know. I would love to be part of any research on hair loss. I also want to let women who are dealing with this out there know that they are not alone. If we band together, maybe something can be done to get more attention for this issue. You can ask any woman who deals with this and I promise that she will agree that this is an emotional roller-coaster of anger, despair, embarrassment, shame, helplessness, and sadness.

Carol's Story

I've been experiencing extreme thinning at the front of the top of my head. I'm only thirty-one. The strange thing is the back and sides of my head itch terribly, and the hair loss increases during the summer when it's hot. Then it gets better in the winter. I saw my internist, and he diagnosed "stress." This is *not* from stress.

Annie's Story

I am forty years old, and my hair loss started when I was thirty-five. I was prepared for wrinkles and other age-related things but not this. I know hair loss is hard on men, but it's harder on women. I know of no other women under the age of sixty with this problem. I feel like a weirdo and I can't talk about it with anyone. My doctor tells me that there are a lot of women like me, but that they all hide it well and it's like a taboo to talk about. He also tells me that there are a lot of other worse things that can happen to me (which is true, I know), but I think that statement is just his cop-out regarding what he calls "my little problem." He doesn't care at all. I am looking for another doctor.

Rachel's Story

I'm fifty-three. Most of my life I've had very long hair and have almost always worn it back, off my face. So I didn't really have an abrupt "awakening" that I was losing my hair until I went to a dermatologist for my rosacea. When he moved my bangs, he suggested that I might have "female pattern baldness." He asked me to ask my husband if he'd noticed my hair thinning. When the doctor said that, I realized that my hairbrush had seemed quite full lately but compared to who else's hairbrush?

Then I started looking at my hair, and I realized that it did feel thinner. My husband agreed. My father and two of my three brothers are balding. My mother had a full head of healthy hair.

I started searching on the Internet for information on female pattern baldness and I was extremely lucky to find a support group on-line where I've been going for about a year. If not for their knowledge and warm, positive encouragement, I don't know what any of us would have done or felt. It is a very lonely feeling for a woman to be losing her hair. A woman's friends and family don't really understand.

I was very lucky. I only had to go to two doctors before I found a fabulous female gynecologist who was eager to help me. I brought her all my Internet research. She told me she has set up a special file for my things and asked me to please not stop bringing her information. She has encouraged me and said that often doctors do not have the time to do this much research. She had been genuinely concerned and has spent a lot of time with me in the office. She has incorporated vitamins and other natural treatments into my hair loss treatment.

My doctor and I are even E-mailing each other with questions and suggestions. She has admitted to me that doctors really do not know very much about hormones. She wrote, "Most doctors learn very little about hormones in medical school or even in residency. All I know I learned from a book on gynecological endocrinology and at continuing education courses. An anti-aging conference recently was the biggest eye-opener of them all."

I gave her a copy of Dr. Lee's book *What Your Doctor May Not Have Told You About Menopause* as a present.

I'm so blown away by this caring doctor I've found. I told her it's like she's from another planet compared to other doctors. I am very grateful to her for all her concern. We are both learning about hair loss together and trying things out. I thought such doctors were a thing of the past, like dinosaurs.

What I've found is that you can't really trust blood tests because the labs are not standardized. This is a stupid thing. We also need to be able to compare our imbalances to the "normal" range. And nobody knows what is normal to whom!

I've found that truer levels of hormones can be measured by a saliva test and that natural hormones in cream form can work better than the pill form because the creams are better absorbed into the bloodstream.

So much is available to help people medically besides synthetic pharmaceutical drugs. Since natural things like herbs or plants can't be patented, the medical industry won't take them as seriously because they can't make the kind of profit off them as they would from synthetic drugs whose patents they can own. I find it extremely offensive to know that greed takes prominence over the health of people. Greed is the great malignant insanity that this country must cure. I think we have become a country of corporations, by corporations, and for corporations.

Why hasn't medical research devoted time to understanding women's health and the workings of hormones? Why is so little known about them? We are half the population who spend our lives taking care of the other half!

Sugar and Hair Loss

I've put this section entirely in this treatments chapter, even though it deals with both a contributing cause to hair loss and the corresponding preventive and treatment diet. That's because sugar imbalance isn't a *primary* cause of hair loss. It is, instead, a strong contributing factor in the hormonal imbalance factors that are at the root (again, pardon that inevitable pun) of most kinds of hair loss.

As you'll recall from The Hormone Connection section in Chapter One, the delicate balance of male and female hormones is crucial to the issue of hair loss and so are the hormones regulated by the thyroid. But another hormone also plays a role in hair loss, and that's *insulin*.

The pancreas creates *insulin* and *glucagon*, which both maintain stable blood-sugar levels. Here's how they work:

• Your body converts food and its nutrients into glucose, a sugar. Insulin helps your body's cells use glucose for fuel, thereby lowering the amount of sugar remaining in your bloodstream.

• Glucagon stimulates your liver to release its stored sugar into the bloodstream when the amount of sugar in the bloodstream needs to be raised.

• These two hormones—insulin and glucagon—play off each other to keep your blood-sugar levels balanced.

Diabetes, a chronically high level of blood sugar, results when the pancreas can't produce enough insulin or the body can't properly use the insulin. In this case, the sugar isn't able to go from the bloodstream to the cells where it's crucially needed to fuel the body, and it's not able to go to the liver to be stored until it's needed for fuel.

Hypoglycemia, or low blood sugar, is the opposite of diabetes. When you have hypoglycemia, your body's sugar is used for fuel by the cells to such an extent that not enough circulates in the bloodstream. This can be caused by not eating often enough for blood-sugar levels to be replenished—giving you the light-headed or queasy feeling you get if you haven't eaten in a few hours or all day—or from too much insulin.

What does all this have to do with hair?

The Relationship Between Insulin and Testosterone

There is an important link between your body's insulin level and its testosterone level. How does your insulin level tie into your testosterone level? An important class of hormones called the *eicosanoids* (pronounced eye-KŌ-sah-noids), which biochemist Barry Sears, Ph.D., author of *The Zone* calls "the molecular glue" that holds the body together, are the master switches that control all human bodily functions. Every system, including the ones that govern how much fat we store in our bodies, a key factor in the action of testosterone, is also controlled by the eicosanoids.

Dr. Sears realized that, if you can control these eicosanoids, you can control virtually every aspect of human physiology. He created *The Zone* diet specifically to balance the eicosanoids.

Using the Insulin-Testosterone Link to Foster Hair Growth

Because of the insulin-testosterone link, by controlling your insulin level you can also control your testosterone level. Through a sugar-balancing diet, you can help regulate your testosterone levels and create an internal physiological environment supportive of hair growth.

Foods affect hormones quickly, anywhere from a few minutes to a few weeks. Scientists already know that diets high in animal fats trigger the release of more testosterone into your bloodstream. Studies have shown that low-fat or vegetarian diets lower levels of testosterone in your bloodstream. A low-fat diet also lowers estrogen levels in both men and women. Have you ever noticed that obese men can have breast enlargement? That's because someone who is overweight, even a man, is more likely to have a higher level of estrogen.

All in all, a high-fat diet throws your normal hormonal balance into a tizzy. And this directly affects your hair loss, since testosterone plays such a pivotal role in androgenetic alopecia and other hormonally triggered forms of hair loss. A high-fat diet also reduces the amount of a protein known as *sex hormone binding globulin,* which keeps a sex hormone inactive until your body needs it. If you have less of this protein in your bloodstream, more testosterone will freely circulate, ready to be converted to hair follicle-killing DHT at the follicle if conditions there are conducive. A high-fat diet also contributes to the conversion of testosterone to DHT in another way: Oil glands in the hair follicle hold 5-alpha reductase, the enzyme that converts testosterone to DHT, and higher amounts of circulating hormones (due to a reduction of sex hormone binding globulin, as explained, including testosterone, can increase oil gland activity. This is compounded by the fact that the oil glands in the hair follicles of balding areas are always larger than the oil glands in the other areas of your scalp that are not balding.

Although Dr. Sears did not mention hair loss in *The Zone,* after reading his book I thought that a sugar-balancing diet low in animal fat and similar to *The Zone* diet—which would control testosterone, insulin, and the eicosanoids—would help prevent and treat hair loss by creating a more favorable hormonal balance and, therefore, lower DHT levels. This kind of a diet would also boost other hair loss preventive measures and treatments.

I spoke with Dr. Sears, and he agreed. "At the molecular level, balding can be viewed as a hormonal disturbance condition," Dr. Sears said. "It is clear that the hormone dihydrotestosterone (DHT), which is a breakdown product of testosterone, is a major contributor to baldness. Therefore, interventions that lower DHT levels should have a beneficial effect on balding." Whether you lower DHT levels by using pharmaceutical drugs, herbal or natural treatments, or diet, the outcome is helpful as both a preventive measure and a treatment.

"Another biochemical approach is modulating the production of testosterone itself," he continued, "which can be accomplished using dietary measures." Dr. Sears explained how a low-fat, sugar-balancing diet does this and how insulin plays a pivotal role. This kind of diet is

> "based on keeping another hormone, insulin, in a tight zone: not too high, not too low. By doing so, one is able to control the body's production of an essential fatty acid called *arachidonic acid*. By controlling the levels of arachidonic acid, the production of testosterone is also controlled."

Although dietary control is always more difficult than simply taking a drug, it also has *no* negative side effects. In fact, controlling arachidonic acid will have some additional benefits, particularly at the level of the hormonal system known as *eicosanoids*, which are superhormones of the body that virtually control all of our physiological systems. Among other things, they control high blood pressure and the synthesis of structural proteins such as keratin, the major structural component of hair.

How do you keep this tricky hormonal balance? Dr. Sears explained that, when you have the right ratio of protein to carbohydrates in your diet, you can control the eicosanoid hormones with druglike precision. In short, he explained, you are treating food as if it were a prescription drug, delivering the right balance of protein and carbohydrates at every meal.

In my experience and in the experience of many other people I've shared this information with and who have implemented this balanced way of eating, the sugar-balancing diet has been effective in helping to control hair loss, especially in combination with herbal or pharmaceutical treatments.

The Sugar-Balancing Diet

To achieve the sugar-balancing effect, Dr. Sears recommends that each meal you eat contain 30 percent protein, 40 percent complex carbohydrates, and 30 percent monounsaturated fats. This is also similar to the diet recommended to diabetics. You can do this easily and with great precision by following the formulas in *The Zone*, which show you how to calculate your own unique protein requirements based on your weight, lean body mass, and activity level.

Here are the general food guidelines for the standard 30-40-30 sugar-balancing diet:

• Protein: Consume lean protein sources, including turkey, chicken, fish, red meat (only occasionally), and soy products.

• Carbohydrates: Include fruits, vegetables, and beans in your meals. Do not eat potatoes, pasta, and bread regularly. They are immediately converted to glucose and disturb insulin levels when your blood sugar rises very quickly and then falls. This is very bad for proper hormonal function and balance.

• Monounsaturated fats: Use only the following oils in their whole form as fruits or nuts or as extracted oils: extra virgin olive, almond, avocado, cashew, macadamia, pecan, hazelnut, and pistachio.

• Alcohol: More than one alcoholic drink per day is not advised. Alcohol plays havoc with your blood sugar levels and your hormones. It robs your body of vital nutrients, including vitamin C, vitamin B, zinc, and folic acid. Alcohol also acts as a diuretic and can cause severe dehydration, which damages all of your systems and directly affects the condition of your scalp and hair growth.

• Caffeine: Limit your caffeine intake. Long-term use of caffeine depletes the body of vitamins B and C and the minerals potassium and zinc. This stresses the adrenal glands, which causes the depletion of vital nutrients in the bloodstream, which then adversely affects DHT levels.

• Nicotine: Avoid nicotine. It depletes the body of many important nutrients, and long-term use puts extreme stress on the adrenal glands.

Physicians commonly offer the following additional guidelines for keeping your blood sugar balanced:

• Eat five or six small meals a day: breakfast, lunch, and dinner, with a light snack between each meal and a nightly snack.

• If you are not overweight, your body will make better use of its insulin. Overweight people are prone to diabetes, which is chronically high blood sugar.

• Don't let more than three hours pass without eating something.

• Avoid refined and processed foods. Whole and natural foods are used by the body more slowly and evenly, which keeps blood sugar levels steady, not spiking or dropping sharply.

• Avoid snacks and desserts that contain refined sugar, such as candy, cakes, cookies, pastries, ice cream, canned fruits, and the like. They cause blood sugar to rise quickly and then drop.

• Soluble fiber, the kind found in vegetables, oats, and fruits, helps your intestines absorb glucose (sugar) steadily and evenly.

• Reducing your salt intake reduces blood-sugar levels.

• Exercise lowers blood-sugar levels.

• Stress can cause fluctuations in blood-sugar levels.

• When your blood sugar is extremely low and you feel dizzy, light-headed, disoriented, or nauseated, drink eight ounces of orange juice. It will raise your blood-sugar level almost immediately and will relieve symptoms in a few minutes. You will begin to feel its effects after just the first few sips of orange juice.

Further Commentary on a Sugar-Balancing Diet

In her critically acclaimed book, *Women's Bodies, Women's Wisdom*, Christiane Northrup, M.D., also discusses the role of sugar and fats in fighting hair loss. In the 1998 revised and updated edition of her book, Dr. Northrup explains that even a subtle hormone imbalance "at the level of the androgen-sensitive hair follicle" can trigger hair loss. These subtle imbalances "do not show up in standard testing," she warns, "and are associated with insulin resistance." Her advice is the same as what I surmised a few years earlier from reading *The Zone* and then discussed with Dr. Sears. "Follow an eicosanoid-balancing diet and lose excess body fat," Dr. Northrup writes.

Androgenetic Alopecia Treatments

Women are in a "Catch-22" position when it comes to drug treatments for androgenetic alopecia. While many drugs may work to some degree for some women, doctors are reluctant to prescribe them, and drug companies aren't exactly falling over themselves to test existing or new drugs specifically for their ability to prevent and treat female pattern baldness. When you hear why, you'll wonder who threw logic out the window: *Women can get pregnant and these drugs shouldn't be used by pregnant women because they can harm the fetus.* Well, guess what? Women shouldn't use *any* medications when they're pregnant, not even an over-the-counter pain reliever like aspirin, let alone a strong pharmaceutical like those prescribed for any number of disorders, but that doesn't stop drug companies or doctors from making these available to women and always with the warning that pregnant women must not take them. Any sensible woman heeds these warnings. They're used to doing so. And yet this fear on the part of the drug companies and physicians is one of the things standing in the way of progress in the treatment of women's hair loss.

A few drugs on the market now are used to treat other conditions but have been shown in a few studies and in clinical experience also to have some effect on women's hair loss. There have been few studies of their effectiveness in treating hair loss, and success rates in producing hair growth vary from 25 percent to 75 percent for the same drugs, depending upon which study you read. What that means is that two different studies of the same drug can show two different levels of effectiveness! Improved study methods and more studies are needed.

What *has* been established, at least regarding the drugs currently on the market, is that treatment needs to be continued for about a year before substantial improvement is shown. That's not as long as it sounds in the world of hair. Remember that hair goes through growth cycles (see Chapter One).

Physicians are reluctant to use systemic treatment (a pill or other form of internal treatment that affects your entire system) unless they know that the hair loss is due to an excess of androgen in the system or a sensitized "over-response" to the so-called "normal" amounts of androgen in the system. That's because these systemic treatments may lower the body's androgen levels.

Therefore, physicians often choose topical treatments (those that are applied directly to the scalp).

The best results from treatment happen when you begin treatment as soon as possible after the hair loss begins because prolonged androgenetic alopecia may destroy many of the hair follicles. The use of anti-androgens after prolonged hair loss will at least help prevent further hair loss and encourage some hair regrowth from those follicles that have been dormant but are still viable. Stopping treatment will result in the hair loss resuming if the androgens aren't kept in check in some other way. Maintaining your vitamin and mineral levels helps while you're on anti-androgen medications.

There are many promising natural treatments available and in research. These are discussed in this section and in Chapter Five, which focuses on research for future treatments.

As always, treatments have the best chance of being effective if they are geared to the cause of the hair loss as well as to triggering hair growth.

Propecia/Proscar

The drug finasteride inhibits the enzyme 5-alpha reductase, thereby inhibiting the production of prostate-harming, follicle-killing DHT. It was first marketed to treat the prostate under the brand name Proscar in 5 mg pills. In 1998, a 1 mg version with the brand name Propecia entered the market as the first pill approved by the FDA for men's hair loss. It works quite well for most men in both preventing hair loss and triggering regrowth, and it may work for some women, although women *must not* take it if they are pregnant and *must not* get pregnant while on the drug because of the risk of birth defects in a male fetus. Less than 2 percent of men experience transient sexual side effects including erectile and libido difficulties. In women these side effects do not occur.

Rogaine

The drug minoxidil was first marketed to treat high blood pressure. In topical lotion form, under the brand name Rogaine, it is approved for the treatment of hair loss in both men and women, and it is available over-the-counter in regular (2 percent) and extra-strength (5 percent). Rogaine can produce regular terminal hair when used as directed. Some patients report that Rogaine is even more effective when it is used in combination with other treatments. (See various additional treatments for women's hair loss in Chapter Two.) Side effects include itchy, flaky scalp and dry mouth. Lowered blood pressure and dizziness are less common side effects. Rogaine is reported to be a bit more effective in women than in men for treating androgenetic alopecia and other types of hair loss.

Tricomin

Manufactured by ProCyte Corp., this topical solution is a copper compound that stimulates hair follicles and prevents healthy follicles from staying in their natural resting phase (the hair shaft's natural fallout phase) for too long and becoming dormant. Available over-the-counter, the solution is applied directly to the scalp. The product's strength is lower than the strength of the solution tested in clinical trials. Therefore, there is no significant data regarding its effectiveness. Tricomin is new on the market for both men and women. There are no significant side effects.

Nizoral/Ketoconazole

Available as a topical treatment by prescription, Ketoconazole is currently used as an antifungal agent in the treatment of fungal infections. It also has anti-androgenic effects and can cause a reduction in the production of testosterone and other androgens by the adrenal gland and by the male and female reproductive organs (in women, the ovaries). Because of this action, it can be used to help treat hair loss. Nizoral shampoo contains 2 percent Ketoconazole and is prescribed not only for the treatment of scalp conditions, but also in combination with other treatments for androgenetic alopecia. A 1 percent version is now available over-the-counter, but it may not be as effective as the 2 percent prescription strength. There are no significant side effects.

Spironolactone

Sold under the brand name Aldactone and Spironolactone, these tablets are prescribed as a diuretic (one that doesn't deplete potassium) in the treatment of mildly high blood pressure and more recently as a very effective treatment for heart failure. It is also used to treat women with androgenetic alopecia because it decreases ovarian and adrenal androgen production and also prevents DHT from binding to androgen receptors. The side effects can include breast tenderness, menstrual irregularities, cramps, diarrhea, and drowsiness. It's not to be taken if you're pregnant. Unless using the drug to treat heart failure, men shouldn't use the drug because of its feminizing effects. A topical form of the drug can also be used, but it can cause irritation to the scalp.

Estrogen/Progesterone

Also known as hormone replacement therapy (HRT) and commonly prescribed at menopause, estrogen and progesterone pills and creams are probably the most common systemic form of treatment for androgenetic alopecia for women in menopause or whose estrogen and/or progesterone are lacking for other reasons.

Cyproterone Acetate

Sold under the brand name Androcur, cyproterone acetate is used to reduce a man's sex drive in cases of excessive sex drive and for the treatment of sexual overaggression. A member of the progestin family of hormones, this drug blocks the binding of DHT to its receptors. Because of this, it can be effective in treating women's androgenetic alopecia and is a popular form of treatment worldwide, especially in Europe. Spironolactone, however, is more commonly prescribed in the United States.

Cyproterone Acetate with Ethinyloestradiol

Sold under the brand name Diane 35 and Diane 50, this contraceptive tablet is prescribed in Europe for women's androgenetic alopecia. The drug works by blocking some of the actions of male hormones commonly present in women. Although it's possible for the drug to stop further hair loss and trigger regrowth of hair within about a year, it needs to be used on an ongoing basis in order to maintain regrowth and eliminate hair loss. Possible side effects include breast tenderness, headaches, and decreased libido. It does have one good side effect—it helps prevent osteoporosis. The drug is a combination of cyproterone and estradiol, an estrogen. Both Diane 35 and Diane 50 contain 2 mg of cyproterone. Diane 35 contains 0.035 mg of estradiol. Diane 50 contains 0.050 mg of estradiol. The drug is as effective as, if not more than, spironolactone. It is not available in the United States, but people are obtaining it via the Internet. (This area is somewhat gray legally because buying via the Internet is so new.)

Dexamethasone

Dexamethasone is sold in the following forms:

- Decadron elixir

- Decadron tablets

- Decaspray topical aerosol

- Dexamethasone elixir

- Dexamethasone tablets

- Dexamethasone solution

Dexamethasone is a synthetic corticosteroid primarily used as an anti-inflammatory to treat various diseases. Because it suppresses androgens in women, it can be effective in treating androgenetic alopecia. High-dose long-term use, as with other corticosteroids, can cause a variety of physical and emotional side effects depending upon how the drug is administered, so discuss these risks with your doctor.

Cimetadine

Sold under the brand named Tagamet, cimetadine is commonly used to reduce acid secretion in the stomach, in stomach and duodenal ulcers, in inflammation of the esophagus, and in other digestive disorders. Since it also has an anti-androgenetic effect by blocking DHT from binding to its receptor, it can be used to treat androgenetic alopecia in women. Men should not use it in high doses needed to treat hair loss because of its feminizing side effects at these high doses.

Flutamide

Sold in capsule form under the brand name Eulexin, this anti-androgen is not part of the steroid family. It is used to treat a variety of androgen-influenced diseases, including prostate cancer. There have been only a few published studies on its effectiveness in treating women's androgenetic alopecia, but they look promising, and in one study, flutamide outdid Spironolactone.

Oral Contraceptive Pills

Since birth control pills decrease the production of ovarian androgens, they can be used to treat women's androgenetic alopecia. Keep in mind, however, that the same cautions must be followed whether a woman takes contraceptive pills solely to prevent contraception or to treat female pattern baldness. For example, smokers over thirty-five who take "the pill" are at higher risk for blood clots and other serious conditions. Discuss your medical and lifestyle history thoroughly with your doctor. Contraceptive pills come in various hormonal formulations, and your doctor can determine which is right for your specific needs, switching pills if necessary until you are physically and emotionally comfortable with the formulation. Note: *Only low androgen index birth control pills should be used to treat hair loss. High androgen index birth control pills actually contribute to hair loss by triggering it or enabling it once it's been triggered by something else.*

Green Tea

Many studies have documented green tea's therapeutic properties, including its ability to act as a powerful antioxidant. Green tea also has been shown to inhibit the androgens that trigger androgenetic alopecia in both men and women. It has been suggested that a minimum of three cups of green tea per day is needed to achieve these effects.

Gamma Linolenic Acid

Studies have shown that unsaturated fatty acids such as gamma linolenic acid (GLA) inhibit the enzyme 5-alpha reductase, which converts testosterone into hair follicle–harming DHT. GLA, one of the essential fatty acids, is found in linseed oil, sunflower oil, black currant oil, evening primrose oil, and soy oil. One teaspoon per day of one of these oils will benefit you in your fight against hair loss. You can use sunflower oil on a salad or take black currant oil or evening primose oil in capsule form. GLA promotes healthy hair, skin, and nails and is an effective anti-inflammatory with none of the side effects of a prescription anti-inflammatory. One 500 mg capsule of black currant oil twice a day should lead to an improvement in hair quality, texture, and density in six to eight weeks.

Zinc

Both studies and clinical experience show that the mineral zinc, alone and in combination with other substances, inhibits the activity of 5-alpha reductase, thereby protecting your hair follicles from DHT. It has been used successfully in the treatment of prostate disorders and baldness. In combination with vitamin B_6 and azelaic acid, the zinc treatment becomes even more effective for treating hair loss. Zinc and azelaic acid are available as a topical treatment.

When taking zinc orally, use only zinc picolinate, which is the best-absorbed form. Your dosages will be based upon the length of time you'll need to stay on the zinc. It is commonly used at 60 mg per day for six months. For longer-term use, your doctor will modify the dosage and give you a schedule. Zinc is available in pills and capsules for oral use. The doctor can also advise you regarding the zinc–vitamin B_6 combination.

Emu Oil

That's right, we're talking about oil from the emu, an Australian bird. Emu oil contains a high level of linolenic acid (see Gamma Linolenic Acid), a potent 5-alpha reductase inhibitor.

Emu oil is used topically on the scalp. Studies and clinical experience show that it helps prevent hair loss and stimulates hair growth and hair follicles. If you don't see this in your health food store, ask if you can order it.

Asian Natural Hair Loss Treatments

The traditional medicines of Asia, in particular of China and Japan, offer effective preventions and treatments for hair loss and general hair health. "In Asian herbal medicine, sesame oil is the one used most often for healing purposes where hair and scalp are concerned," reports author Michelle Dominique Leigh in *Inner Peace, Outer Beauty*, her book of traditional Japanese natural treatments for skin and hair. Among those her research singles out are the following:

Sesame Oil Treatment

Sesame oil is used to prevent hair loss, nourish hair and scalp, heal, and moisturize. Use once a week.

• Before shampooing, apply sesame oil (pure, not blended with other oils) to slightly moistened hair.

• Massage scalp thoroughly, oiling the hair all the way to the ends.

• Wrap your head in a warm towel and leave the oil treatment on for at least thirty minutes or as long as three hours.

• Rinse with very warm water.

• Shampoo well and rinse.

Sesame Oil and Ginger Scalp Treatment

This treatment is used to stimulate hair growth, remedy falling hair, heal scalp irritations, and activate circulation. Because of ginger's strength, it is not recommended for sensitive scalps. Use three times per week as a prolonged remedy.

• Grate a piece of gingerroot with a ginger grater. Squeeze the ginger through a piece of gauze, catching the juice in a bowl. Discard the ginger pieces and mix the ginger juice in a one-to-one ratio with pure sesame oil, beating well with a whisk. Prepare it fresh for each use.

• Use the solution as a massage oil for the scalp, rubbing it into the scalp and the root end of hair for ten minutes. Shampoo and rinse.

• You may also leave the treatment on your head for a few more minutes before washing. Some scalps may become irritated by ginger. If you feel any stinging sensation, wash the oil out immediately and decrease the amount of ginger in future treatments.

Garlic Hair Loss Treatment

Garlic has been used consistently since ancient times by many cultures throughout the world, and modern science can attest to its healing properties. It has long been used by Japanese women to treat hair loss. Thankfully, we no longer have to bear the pungent smell of garlic in such treatments since odorless garlic oil, widely available in gelatin capsules, can be substituted for fresh garlic. Leigh suggests the following treatment. It is done on a dry scalp, once a day for at least three months.

• Warm the affected area with a steamed towel.

• Apply the garlic oil to the thinning or bald scalp areas.

• Gently massage the oil into the scalp for a minute. Blot the excess oil but leave the garlic coating on the scalp.

• You may want to do this in the evenings and then place a towel on your pillow at bedtime. In the morning, shampoo and rinse.

Alopecia Areata Treatments

Because the causes of alopecia areata (and universalis and totalis) are not known, treatments are based on current speculation regarding the immune system. As you read in Chapter One, what scientists *do* know is that, in patients with alopecia areata, there is an immune system response at the hair follicles, which are attacked by the system as if the follicles were invading foreign bodies. What scientists do *not* know yet is whether the immune system is responding to something as yet undiscovered around the follicles or to the follicles themselves and why. Therefore, the best that can be done to treat alopecia areata with drugs is to use a drug's ability to influence the immune system in some way. Researchers and doctors admit that these treatments are merely shots in the dark and that they have wildly variable response rates. Since alopecia areata often goes into spontaneous remission—and hair starts growing again, even without treatment— there is *always* hope.

Natural treatments have also been effective in treating alopecia areata. Some of these treatments are based on how they affect the immune system and some are not. While it may be a mystery why some of them work, studies and clinical experience show that in many cases they do work and usually with far fewer side effects than pharmaceutical drugs have.

Keep in mind the following facts about treating alopecia areata:

• If you have had bald patches for less than one year, you are more likely to respond to treatment, and your success rate using treatment is about 75 percent.

• If you have had alopecia areata for more than two years, whether you've had treatment or not, you are less likely to respond to treatment.

• Forty percent of those who have long-term hair loss due to alopecia areata will respond to treatment.

• Everyone with alopecia areata may be able to regrow their hair even after many years of hair loss. Spontaneous regrowth at any time is possible.

• At this time, there is no permanent cure and no universally proven therapy for inducing remission.

• A range of therapies can bring partial success, but when treatment is stopped, the alopecia areata returns in many patients. Unfortunately, there's always a chance that the disease will return even during treatment. In other patients, treatment triggers a remission, and alopecia does not return for a while or ever. Remissions can even be permanent.

Confused? Well, so is everyone studying, treating, or suffering from alopecia areata. What it all boils down to is this: Your hair may come back if you use one or any number of treatments, but, then again, it may not. It may come back for a while and then fall out again. Or it may come back and never fall out again. If you don't treat alopecia areata, your hair may not regrow in the bald patches, it may get worse and you'll lose even more from existing or new patches, or it may all grow back either temporarily or permanently.

Yes, I know that all of this sounds crazy, but unfortunately it's where alopecia areata stands right now. And that's why genetics researcher Dr. Angela Christiano, who discovered the first gene linked to hair loss, calls this form of hair loss "the madness that is alopecia areata."

Pharmaceutical Treatments

Corticosteroids

Cortisone and similar drugs are applied topically in cream or lotion form or injected into and around the balding area. This is the most popular treatment for alopecia areata and is most effective when treatment begins within the first year of the onset of hair loss. In usual low doses, side effects are mild and include irritation, acne, and atrophy of the skin around the treatment site, particularly if the treatment is delivered by injection. High doses of topical corticosteroids can bring on some of the same side effects as when the drug is taken orally because of the possibility of systemic absorption.

Dithranol

This tarlike ointment that's applied to the scalp is commonly used to treat psoriasis and is also used to treat mild or early stages of alopecia areata. Like other treatments, its success rate is variable.

Minoxidil

Sold under the brand name Rogaine, this topical solution is also used to treat androgenetic alopecia, also known as *male* or *female pattern baldness*. It is sometimes temporarily effective in mild cases of alopecia areata.

Systemic Cortisone

Taken internally in pill form, cortisone and other corticosteroids are far more powerful than when applied topically or injected at hair loss sites. However, they are also more dangerous. For this reason, a systemic application (meaning that it affects your entire system, not just one local area) of this drug can only be used for a short time and only in advanced cases of alopecia areata when all other treatment methods have failed. Side effects of systemic use can be quite serious and include weight gain, acne, menstrual problems, mood swings, migraines, eye complications, osteoporosis, high blood pressure, diabetes, and stunted growth when taken by children.

PUVA

Puva is the combination of 8-mop and ultraviolet light. The chemical 8-methoxysporalen (8-mop), an irritant that also modulates the body's immune response, is applied to the scalp, and then the scalp is exposed to uva, long-wave ultraviolet light. Treatments are typically given two to three times per week for three to six weeks. This treatment is used by some doctors as a last resort and not at all by others. Studies show that about half of those patients with mild alopecia areata show some response to the treatment and then only when they receive extensive treatment involving light exposure to the entire body, not just the balding sites.

Irritants

Irritants or allergens are applied to the scalp in order to cause an immune response in the hopes of luring the immune system's "fighting force" away from the hair follicles and to the top of the scalp to battle the dermatitis (inflammation) and allergic reaction caused by the irritants. Theoretically, this leaves the follicles free from immune attack for a while so that they can grow hair again. The problem is that the fighting team at the follicles may not be the same force the immune system calls upon to fight the irritants at the scalp. Results, therefore, from the use of irritants are wildly variable. Because the whole purpose of using these chemicals is to irritate the scalp or bring upon an allergic reaction, this form of treatment can be very uncomfortable, causing irritation, rash, and itching. Side effects include an extreme version of these three plus swollen lymph nodes, hives, and a change in skin pigmentation at the treatment site.

Cyclosporin

Cyclosporin is an immunosuppressive drug that is used to stop the immune system from attacking transplanted organs after transplant surgery. It works by slowing down the immune system to the point where it is barely functioning. Using cyclosporin or any other immunosuppressive drug to treat alopecia areata is like dropping an atomic bomb to kill a fly. These drugs are life threatening because they leave the body without protection and at extremely high risk to infection that can be fatal, as well as to kidney dysfunction. Because of these extreme risks, doctors use cyclosporin and other drugs of this class only in alopecia areata experimental research and not in routine treatment.

Natural Treatments

Basic Essential Oil Treatment

Created by Melanie Von Zabuesnig to treat her own long-term alopecia areata, which had progressed to almost total baldness, this formula restored her hair within six months. It was printed in *Natural Health* magazine after the magazine ran an article she wrote detailing her successful treatment.

Essential oils are potent and have documented, researched medical properties. They must be handled carefully and never applied to the skin without first being blended into a base oil.

Melanie Von Zabuesnig now devotes her time to providing customized formulas for hair loss patients, according to the type and extent of hair loss, age, and scalp condition. See the Resource Guide under Essential Oil Treatment for information on how to contact her.

The following formula is her basic essential oil treatment for alopecia areata:

1. Add to two teaspoons of jojoba oil the following essential oils:
   - nine drops of rosemary essential oil
   - six drops of lavender essential oil

2. Mix and then thoroughly massage into the scalp and leave on overnight.

3. In the morning, rinse, alternating between hot and cold water.

Note: Rosemary should not be used by children under five, pregnant women, or those with high blood pressure, diabetes, or epilepsy.

To enhance this treatment, in the morning after rinsing off the basic essential oil treatment, massage a half teaspoon of cayenne extract into the scalp with a soft toothbrush. Leave the mixture on for fifteen minutes and then rinse, alternating between hot and cold water. Do not use this solution on small children or sensitive scalps. Don't let the cayenne water drip into your eyes or face when rinsing, as it will burn.

Aloe Vera

Because of aloe vera's healing and anti-inflammatory properties, some people use 100 percent aloe vera gel (either directly from the plant or bottled). Studies show that it stimulates the immune system, acts as an antiviral, and contains natural substances that are implicated in hair growth stimulation. It can be effective in treating psoriasis, male and female pattern baldness, and alopecia areata.

Stress Reduction (Meditation, Massage, Acupuncture)

It has long been theorized that stress may trigger or exacerbate alopecia areata, and there have been clinical examples of remission as an outcome of stress-reduction methods. Meditation and massage also help by reducing stress. Studies have also pointed to possible reduction of stress through acupuncture treatments for alopecia areata.

Sunlight

Studies have suggested that sunlight can trigger the body's healing mechanisms and affect the immune system. Ultraviolet light (which comes from the full spectrum of light provided by the sun) is used to treat alopecia areata. Many alopecia areata patients report that direct exposure to sunlight from special lights in a clinical setting has helped hair regrow.

Zinc

Zinc is used in the treatment of androgenetic alopecia and may also be of benefit in treating alopecia areata. Several studies conducted in Europe show that people with alopecia areata have a zinc deficiency. Anyone wishing to try zinc should do so under the guidance of a physician who can prescribe the proper dosages since zinc can be toxic at high dosages.

Chinese Herbs

Chinese herbs have long been used to treat all forms of hair loss, including alopecia areata. One of the most potent herbs is called Ho Shou Wu, which literally translates to "Mr. Ho has black hair." The herb can be found in Chinese herbal shops and natural health stores in both capsule and tea form.

Gamma Linolenic Acid (GLA) in Specific Oils

Studies and clinical experience show that essential fatty acids, the active ingredients in certain oils rich in GLA, are effective against the processes that cause not only male and female pattern baldness, but also alopecia areata. These oils include sunflower oil, black currant oil, evening primrose oil, soy oil, and linseed oil. One teaspoon per day of one of these oils is all you'll need. You can take black currant oil or evening primrose oil in capsules or just use one teaspoon of sunflower oil in a salad dressing. By taking just one 500 mg capsule of black currant oil twice per day, you may notice an improvement in the quality of your hair within six to eight weeks. It also works to slow down hair loss and help trigger hair regrowth in balding areas.

Omega 3 Fatty Acids Found in Oils

Oils that are high in omega 3 fatty acids include flaxseed oil, linseed oil, and fish oil. In studies and clinical experience, omega 3 has been shown to benefit in the treatment of cancer, rheumatoid arthritis, systemic lupus, Alzheimer's disease, autoimmune conditions, ulcerative colitis, and other conditions. Because of its anti-inflammatory effect, it also promotes the health of the hair follicles and hair. These oils can be incorporated into your diet and taken in capsule form.

Panel Commentary on Treatments

Dr. Marty Sawaya

• "Pharmaceutical companies don't want cures, they want something that can continuously make them money."

Dr. Ken Washenik

• "A lot of doctors and researchers say that women get facial hair because they are being sloppy while applying Rogaine and it's running onto the face. This is false. We know this is false because the facial hair that's growing is symmetrical, and also if Rogaine *did* grow hair just by dripping on your skin . . . We wish it worked that well! The same androgen problem that causes androgenetic alopecia in women is also responsible for excess facial hair."

• "It makes total sense that Propecia (finasteride) should work in women, but I have not seen the startling improvements in women taking it that I have seen in men. That may be because with women you don't have a nice balding spot to look at, and it's not as easy to tell if there is a lot of hair regrowth."

3

Hair Transplantation

First, do no harm.
—Hippocrates (from the Hippocratic oath,
which all physicians take)

The men's hair transplantation industry has been notorious for being unscrupulous since its beginning. Now those physicians who are opportunists see further opportunity in taking advantage of women as well.

Most people, whether men or women, are not aware of the scope and pitfalls of hair transplantation. While some patients may understand the medical basics of the procedure, few realize the extremely high level of aesthetics and artistry required of this very demanding and exacting cosmetic procedure. Unfortunately, many of the doctors who perform these procedures are as ill informed as their patients and have entered this unregulated specialty either poorly trained and not open to its recent improvements or purely for the money or both.

Slick marketing and high-pressure sales techniques abound in the industry. Yes, it's considered an *industry*. Hair transplantation is handled not so much as the *medical specialty* that it is, one that cares for *patients*, but as a profiteering business that takes aim at potential *consumers*. Not unlike the methods used by car salesmen, the marketing methods of many of the doctors in this field specifically set out to mislead the prospective patient, which is easy to do since the patient is filled with a mixture of hope and desperation about her hair loss.

There are thousands of doctors performing many kinds of transplantation procedures in the country, but there are, quite literally, only a handful who perform these procedures well and to safe, nondisfiguring, state-of-the-art specifications. These talented, ethical, and pioneering few are the conscience of the hair transplantation "industry," and have been speaking up about the problems plaguing it. You will meet a few of them in this chapter and find a list of recommended transplant physicians in the Resource Guide at the end of the book.

Since transplantation is a good option for nearly 90 percent of the balding men in this country, women think that they will make good transplant candidates as well, but this is usually *not* the case. Very few women have the type of hair loss that would make them good candidates, and that's because most women have what's called *diffuse* hair loss. That means that they have an overall thinning in all areas of the head, including the sides and back, the *permanent wreath* areas (as they're called in men) that act as donor sites. It is from these sites that the hair is removed for transplantation to other areas of the head. In men, the donor sites are called *stable* sites, which means that the hair and follicles there are not affected by the DHT that shrinks follicles elsewhere on the head in those with androgenetic alopecia, or what's commonly called *male pattern baldness*. In female pattern baldness, however, these donor areas are usually *unstable*. They are thinning, just like the other areas of the head. The donor areas in women *are* affected by follicle-killing DHT. That means that if you remove hair and accompanying follicles from these donor areas in women and transplant them to other areas, it's just going to fall out. Any doctor who would attempt to transplant hair from an unstable donor site is unethical and just trying to take economic advantage of the patient.

Another difference between male and female pattern baldness is the frontal hairline. Unlike men, women experiencing hair loss still tend to keep their frontal hairline. They don't have to worry about needing a transplant to frame their face and are instead more concerned about loss of volume from the top and back. Transplantation, though, doesn't do much to increase volume. It just moves hair from one place to another. (If you *do* have hair loss in the frontal hairline but you have a stable donor area on the sides or back, you *would* be a good candidate for hair transplantation because you'd be placing hair in a limited thinning area as opposed to seeking overall volume throughout the head. If you have a thinning crown but a stable donor area, you might also make a good transplant candidate.)

The hair transplantation field is at an important crossroads as the general public learns more about the industry's troubles. "The history of this industry has been less than forthcoming and open in its representation of the results obtained from the various hair-restoration procedures over the last thirty-plus years," says Dr. William R. Rassman. In 1995, in the *International Journal of Aesthetic and Restorative Surgery*, Rassman, with his colleague Dr. Robert M. Bernstein, introduced follicular transplantation, the state-of-the-art technique now considered the safest, most natural-looking and medically and cosmetically successful hair transplantation method. Rassman and Bernstein, through their breakthrough adaptation of this technique, their published reports in medical journals, and their outspoken presentations at medical conferences, have emerged as the field's visionaries and consciences. "Much of the lack of openness still exists," Rassman continues. "For this reason, you should be wary of dubious medical claims and results that do not allow direct examination by meeting and examining patients directly. The more primitive techniques of the past will hopefully be laid to rest sooner rather than later."

As a consumer/patient advocate, I speak with both men and women in various stages of the hair loss process, including those who have already undergone hair restoration surgery. Unless they have had state-of-the-art follicular transplantation, most of these people are unhappy with the results, and many even feel that they have been deformed (and, unfortunately, they are often right) by outdated surgical procedures still being performed by lazy, unscrupulous doctors. Later in this chapter, we'll go step-by-step through state-of-the-art follicular transplantation, the preferred method by today's standards. I'll also guide you through outdated procedures that you will want to avoid.

"Hair restoration surgery is the single most common cosmetic surgical procedure performed in men in the United States and is still growing at a substantial rate," Bernstein and Rassman reported in the medical journal *Dermatologic Surgery* in 1997. "Of all cosmetic procedures in men, hair restoration surgery has the potential to produce the most dramatic change in one's appearance. However, in no other form of cosmetic surgery has the road to achieving a desired result been more difficult for the patient. Problems produced by earlier surgical procedures which resulted in partial, incomplete, or distorted appearances over multiple-staged sessions often outweighed the long-term benefits."

It has been a long road to acceptable, natural-looking transplants. "The protracted course of traditional transplant surgeries that included 2 to 5 mm grafts, scalp reductions, or flaps, used alone or in combination, often produced significant disfigurement," Bernstein and Rassman noted. "By using follicular units exclusively in the transplants, the surgeon can safely move large quantities of implants. . . . and can create hair patterns that most closely mimic nature."

Dr. Richard C. Shiell of Melbourne, Australia, applauded Bernstein's and Rassman's advances. "There is no doubt that their techniques are revolutionizing hair restoration surgery," he wrote in *Dermatologic Surgery*, "and almost every practitioner in the field has already been influenced by their past writings and very convincing case presentations."

Despite such major advances in technique, many doctors continue to perform outdated, unacceptable procedures that leave their patients with the pluggy, doll-hair look or worse. Dr. Rassman explains that this "issue is really one of change and the economics of this change. Change does not come easily to the established hair transplanters, but the results of traditional hair transplants have been so bad and so unnatural that the poor unfortunate patients who have received them have been unable to lead normal lives. The harm created from traditional transplantation techniques is the issue, and to argue it one must be blind. Perpetuating the present standard of care which produces substandard results defies logic and undermines our integrity as physicians."

Sadly, some physicians are reluctant to embrace recent procedural advances because they take great skill and training. "For those doctors who do not get good results, the focus should be on how to achieve them, or one should abandon performing the procedure altogether," says Rassman. "Our patients demonstrate a standard which we feel should become the standard of care. This is not a Rassman standard. It is nature's standard. Hair grows in units consisting of one to four hairs each and they should be transplanted that way."

An ideal hair transplant, whether it's performed on a man or a woman, consists of follicular units placed closely together. Hybrid grafting and blend grafting are different names for a two-technique process in which larger grafts are used for the majority of the transplanted area, while the tiny, natural groups of follicular units are used only for the very visible front of the hairline. This technique is *not* recommended, as results are not as natural as those of using just follicular units, and often hairs in the larger grafts do not grow once transplanted.

"It seems that anyone who declares themselves hair transplant specialists seems to be able to promote themselves to a vulnerable and naive public, even with little experience or training in the area," Dr. Rassman cautioned in the July 1994 issue of *Hair Transplant Forum International*, the official publication of the International Society of Hair Restoration Surgery. "Moving from the standard hair transplant quantities with larger grafts to very large quantities of very *small* grafts is a significantly more complex and intricate process than most practitioners realize."

The information on surgical techniques provided in this chapter is the most up-to-date and state-of-the art. The techniques recommended here will give a most natural appearance with no deformities, scarring, pluggy appearance, or cobblestoning. This chapter highlights the work of the two physicians who are considered the voice and conscience of this completely unregulated industry. I have researched Dr. Bernstein's and Dr. Rassman's groundbreaking follicular transplant techniques and interviewed countless physicians. As Dr. O'Tar Norwood (famed for the Norwood Scale, which decades ago set the standard for measuring male pattern baldness) wrote in the May 1997 issue of *Hair Transplant Forum International*, Bernstein's and Rassman's methodology is "an idea whose time has come."

Hair transplantation for both men and women should be completely undetectable and natural looking. I strongly urge anyone who is considering hair transplantation surgery to consider physicians recommended in the Resource Guide at the end of the book and those physicians they may recommend.

Understanding Hair Transplants

As in the case of any other medical procedure, the more you know, the better off you'll be. Gone are the days when people willingly remained in the dark about their own bodies, their treatments, and conditions. An educated and informed person now becomes an active partner in her own health care, which not only leads to better health but also is of great advantage to her doctors since nobody knows her body better than she does.

We'll go step-by-step through the hair transplant procedure, discussing state-of-the-art follicular transplantation as well as the outdated and potentially harmful methods you'll want to avoid. The following questions and answers will prepare you to understand the procedure and methods:

Whose hair will be transplanted onto my head? Does this work like organ transplants where there's a donor and a recipient?

Unlike the case of organ transplants, in a hair transplant *you* are your *own* donor. If you received hair, follicle, and tissue from someone else (other than an identical twin), your body would reject them without immune-suppressant drugs. You donate your hair from what are called your *donor sites*.

Where are my donor sites?

Male pattern baldness and *female pattern baldness* are terms that include the word *pattern*. That's because there is a pattern to the baldness. You've probably noticed, especially in men, that no matter how much hair they lose in the front, top, and crown areas of their heads, the sides and backs of their heads retain hair and sometimes a great deal of it. The sides and back are far less affected by the action of DHT upon their hair follicles. These areas are the donor sites from which the hair you donate to yourself is removed, along with the follicles and some surrounding tissue.

Does the amount of donor hair I have determine how good a candidate I would be for hair transplantation?

Absolutely! It is perhaps the most important of the criteria used to determine whether you can have a successful transplant and benefit from the procedure. If you are among the many women whose androgenetic alopecia—pattern baldness— doesn't follow the pattern that leaves you with thicker hair in the sides and back donor areas, you will not be a good candidate for hair transplantation. Many such women have hair loss of similar degree all over their heads, including the sides and back. This diffuse hair loss takes as much of a toll on the donor sites as on the "pattern" areas. This kind of diffuse baldness is common among women with androgenetic alopecia but much less common among men. If you do not have this diffuse hair loss but just naturally have very thin hair, then the quantity of hair in your donor areas is still not high enough for use in transplantation. Remember that the hair, follicles, and tissue removed from donor areas is gone from there forever. Nevertheless, this removal *doesn't* leave you with gaping bald spots in your donor area, so don't worry. The areas around the donor sites are stitched together, and you should never see any difference.

Where does the surgeon put my donor hair during the transplantation?

Once it's been extracted, it is transplanted to the balding parts of your scalp, into tiny slits that the doctor has created with his or her surgical tools. The donated hair, hair follicles, surrounding tissue, and skin are called *grafts*, and each graft contains one or more hair follicles (ideally no more than four), with accompanying hair, tissue, and skin. In the rest of the chapter, we will go through the entire procedure, step-by-step. No two heads are alike, and you will see that the art of hair transplantation is just as important as its science or medical aspects.

Some people have naturally thick hair, and some don't. How does this factor into your ability to have a successful hair transplant?

Hair density is the number of hair follicles you have per square centimeter of scalp. Scalp laxity is the flexibility and looseness of your scalp. More grafts of hair can be transplanted when your density is high and your scalp laxity is high.

How does the direction in which your hair naturally grows affect hair transplantation?

Your hair doesn't all grow in just one direction. It grows in different directions on different areas of your head. It grows forward at the front and top, down (or away) from the middle of the head on the sides, and back and down in the back of your head. Hair must be transplanted so that it will grow in the proper direction for the new area it will now be growing in.

How do the characteristics of your hair affect hair transplantation?

Coarse hair is bulkier and can therefore be transplanted using fewer hairs per graft since it gives more coverage of the scalp. *Fine hair* has less bulk and can give a very natural look but less coverage than coarser hair. *Wavy and curly hair* lends itself to good visual results in transplantation because a single wavy or curly hair curls on itself and can therefore cover more scalp area than can a straight hair. Curly hair also rises from the scalp and holds its shape (you know how hard it can be to straighten wavy or curly hair!), and these factors also give the appearance of greater coverage. *Straight hair* lies flat against your scalp and gives a less dense appearance in coverage.

Does hair color or skin color play a role in hair transplantation?

The closer your hair color is to your skin color, the better the appearance of the hair's coverage. African hair is dark and very curly and therefore provides the least contrast against various shades of dark skin, giving the best visual hair transplant results. On the opposite end of the spectrum, fair-haired people with a fair complexion also have little contrast between hair and skin shades and also achieve excellent visual hair transplant results. From a visual point of view, people with dark, straight hair and a light complexion pose the most artistic challenges in hair transplantation because they have the most contrast between their hair and skin shades.

What are some of the other visual considerations?

When designing your procedure, your doctor must keep in mind your future hair loss pattern and the rate of that potential hair loss. The design of your restored hairline is crucial. Natural front hairlines vary in shape and density from person to person. Your doctor will choose the recipient sites for the transplanted hair based upon an overall design that may take more than one transplant session to achieve. These sessions typically take place months or even years apart, depending upon the progression of your hair loss.

How soon can a transplant be performed? Can I do it when I'm just beginning to experience hair loss?

In men, doctors can begin transplanting hair in the early stages of hair loss, when their hair is just beginning to recede. Some women may be able to have early transplants, too, depending upon what is causing their hair loss. Unlike men's hair loss, women's hair loss can be stopped (and natural regrowth may be stimulated) in some cases when the underlying cause is treated. Situations in which underlying causes may be treated include a hormonal imbalance due to the use of birth control pills, pregnancy, menopause, or a thyroid condition, or other medical cause. Stress and poor diet also may contribute to reversible hair loss.

How do doctors decide which part of my head will receive the transplanted hair?

The front and top of your head will receive transplanted hair first if needed because these are the areas that frame your face and make the most impact on your appearance. The crown is usually the last area to receive hair (in later procedures), unless it's your only balding area.

How many procedures will I need?

The number of procedures depends upon the extent of your hair loss, the projected hair loss rate, the amount of donor hair you can spare, and other artistic and medical considerations. Men can often have the results they're looking for in just one or two long transplant sessions in which thousands of hairs are transplanted in follicular units of one to four hairs each. Women need more sessions to achieve proper hair density. These sessions can last between five and ten hours each. Future sessions can follow if necessary.

What should I expect during my first meeting with a hair transplant surgeon?

During your first consultation, the doctor should examine your head thoroughly and take a detailed medical history. The examination of your head should include the use of an instrument called the Hair Densitometer.™ This measures your hair density and allows your doctor to properly evaluate the number of hairs in each of your naturally occurring follicular units and the hair loss pattern you may experience over time if it is applicable to your type of hair loss. This instrument compares fine hairs to thick ones, measuring the degree of miniaturization of your hair strands caused by shrinking hair follicles, the progressive diminishing of each hair's diameter and length. Your doctor should put into writing your transplant design and an estimated timeline for any procedures that may be necessary. The doctor should also explain the entire transplant procedure, including any associated risks, and tell you what you can expect in the months following the procedure.

State-of-the-Art Follicular Transplantation

Hair grows in natural clusters of one to four hairs each. These clusters were named *follicular units* by pathologist John Headington in 1984. His observations revolutionized the theoretical approach to hair transplantation. During the late 1980s, another physician made a new approach possible in practice as well as theory: Dr. Bobby L. Limmer of San Antonio, Texas, introduced the microscope into hair transplantation. Physicians were suddenly able to carefully dissect intact follicular units (as well as minigrafts and micrografts) and ready them for transplantation into a patient's recipient sites. Without the aid of the microscope such dissection was nearly impossible, usually destroying the tiny, delicate units.

The stage was now set for further refinement of the transplantation process and a major breakthrough: Robert M. Bernstein, M.D., assistant clinical professor of dermatology at the College of Physicians and Surgeons of Columbia University in New York and a practicing physician performing hair transplants, suggested that for the entire hair transplant procedure only these naturally occurring follicular units should be used and not the larger groupings of hair that weren't follicular units and that contributed to the doll-hair appearance of most hair transplants. Bernstein and his colleague, William R. Rassman, M.D. (an innovative Los Angeles surgeon and the inventor and holder of numerous patents in biotechnology, including the Hair Densitometer which measures hair density), then decided that these follicular units shouldn't be broken apart during the transplantation procedure but should instead be used in their naturally occurring one-, two-, three-, and four-hair groups.

In 1995, Bernstein and Rassman refined the procedure, Bernstein named it *follicular transplantation*, and the two introduced it in the *International Journal of Aesthetic and Restorative Surgery* (vol. 3, no. 2), calling it

> "the logical end point of over thirty years of evolution in hair-restoration surgery, beginning with the traditional large plugs and culminating in the movement of one-, two-, and three-hair units, which mirror the way hair grows in nature. . . . The key to follicular transplantation is to identify the

patient's natural hair groupings, dissect the follicular units from the surrounding skin, and place these units in the recipient site in a density and distribution appropriate for a mature individual."

As mentioned, before the development of follicular transplantation, hair transplants were performed by placing groups of hair in large plugs (of up to twenty hairs each!) into each slit. The result was neither cosmetically pleasing nor natural appearing because hair doesn't naturally sprout from our heads in large plugs.

Bernstein's and Rassman's follicular transplantation also solved many other medical and aesthetic problems associated with previous transplantation methods.

"The critical elements of follicular transplantation are an accurate estimation of the donor supply of hair, meticulous dissection of the follicular units, careful design of the recipient area to maximize the cosmetic impact of the transplant, the use of large numbers of implants in fewer rather than more sessions, a long-term master plan that accounts for the progression of the male pattern alopecia, and realistic expectations on the part of the patient," they reported.

Dr. Rassman stressed that mirroring nature is the key.

"Hair emerges from the scalp in naturally occurring groups called *follicular units*. The surgeon can create hair patterns the way they grow in nature," he wrote. "Once transplanted, these small grafts are often indistinguishable from the natural groups of hair growing in adjacent areas of the scalp."

The difference between older transplant procedures and follicular transplantation, which is state of the art today, is "the size and configuration" of the grafts, said Rassman. And from a visual point of view "this difference is as dramatic as day and night."

Before follicular transplantation and its use of one to four hairs in their naturally occurring clusters, grafts were much larger and classified as *standard grafts*, *minigrafts*, and *micro-*

grafts. None mimic the way hair naturally grows from the head and, unfortunately, all three are still used by many doctors in transplantation procedures.

Standard grafts are those large plugs of hair that give the horrendous doll-hair look, range from 3 to 4 mm in diameter each, and contain twelve to twenty or more hairs per graft or "plug."

Minigrafts are a bit of an improvement over standard grafts but still contribute to the pluggy look, since each graft ranges from 1.2 to 2.5 mm in diameter and contains five to nine hairs.

Micrografts are a big improvement but still less desirable than today's state-of-the-art follicular unit method. Micrografts range in size from 1.0 to 1.5 mm in diameter. Although they only contain one to three hairs per graft, they are not created from natural arrangements of hair strands and their accompanying follicles. The naturally occurring follicular units are ignored by the micrograft method and are "broken apart, and the subsequent damage to many follicles caused a high growth failure rate" after transplantation, Rassman explained.

The Follicular Transplantation Procedure Step-by-Step

A hair transplantation surgery session takes many hours, but it is safely performed in the doctor's office. The doctor is assisted by a team of medical technicians and nurses who each play a highly specialized role in the procedure.

During the procedure you shouldn't feel any pain. First you will be given a mild sedative and then injections in your scalp that will numb the donor and recipient areas. These injections are similar to the novocaine shots the dentist gives you.

During the entire procedure, you will either be in a reclining chair or lying down. As the doctor will tell you before your surgery, you'll be able to listen to music or chat with the medical staff if you'd like during the lengthy transplant session.

After you've received the local anesthesia, the follicular transplantation procedure begins:

1. The doctor chooses a strip of donor hair. Hair on that
   strip is cut short, and then, using a scalpel, the doctor
   removes the strip of scalp from the donor area, which will
   be on the side or back of your head. The donor strip is
   placed in a container filled with a chilled saline solution
   or a special fluid called *Ringer's lactate.*

2. The donor area is stitched closed. This is very important:
   During your initial consultation with the doctor, ask if he
   or she stitches the donor area closed. If the doctor tells you
   that he or she doesn't do that, find another doctor. Do *not*
   use a doctor who leaves the donor site open. An open
   wound, no matter how large or small, greatly increases the
   chances of scarring. Don't worry about how the donor
   area will look after surgery. Hair above the donor site will
   help cover the stitched donor area and the site will heal
   within a week or two. The doctor will then remove the
   stitches, unless dissolvable stitches have been used. With
   no complications, you will have a fine scar that's nearly
   impossible to see and is covered by the surrounding hair.

3. Medical technicians dissect the strip of donor hair under
   a microscope and also trim off extra fatty tissue. Since this
   is a long and exacting part of the procedure, parts of the
   donor strip are placed in a refrigerator set at 40°F while
   other parts of the strip are being dissected and then
   implanted in your recipient sites. During this dissection,
   the donor scalp is cut into follicular units of one to four
   hairs each. You'll remember that these are the naturally
   occurring individual hair clusters. Each unit (whether it's
   a one-hair, two-hair, three-hair, or four-hair unit) includes

the hair strand(s), the hair follicle(s), and some of the surrounding tissue and skin. Great care must be taken not to damage the follicles.

4. During the procedure, your doctor draws on your scalp the outline of the area receiving the transplants. The overall recipient site—the area of your scalp that will receive the transplants during surgery—will have already been chosen during a presurgery exam.

5. Each individual site within the overall area is prepared to receive the transplant graft. A very small slit is created for each with a small, specialized scalpel.

6. The follicular unit hair grafts are placed into the recipient sites in the proper direction of natural hair growth.

After the Transplant

You'll remember that the transplanted hairs are trimmed very short during the procedure. These hairs, of course, are transplanted along with their follicles, and now it's time for the follicles to do their work in their new home. Think of the follicles as your hair factories. They make hair that sprouts from your scalp and grows longer and longer according to the body's natural hair growth cycles. These hairs also fall out, to be replaced by new ones. In people suffering from hair loss, the follicles are unable to produce new hairs of proper size and length and ultimately cannot produce any new hairs at all. The hair-producing follicles that have been transplanted into your recipient sites are healthy follicles that will create new terminal hair strands. But first, those trimmed hairs in your newly situated follicles will fall out. This phenomenon called *shock fallout,* may also affect any original nontransplanted hairs within the recipient areas.

Do not panic when the hair falls out. This is just part of the follicle's natural cycle, and in many cases your original hair as well as your newly transplanted hair will return in a normal growth cycle. Keep the following facts in mind while you wait:

• The normal follicular growth cycle is variable.

• In most people, most of their transplanted hair begins to grow about three to four months after surgery. Additional hair appears over the next several months.

• In a small percentage of people, new growth of most of the hair begins about four to eight months after surgery, with additional hair occasionally appearing up to eighteen months after transplant surgery.

• Hair growth is not constant; it naturally includes a few weeks or even months of inactivity between growth spurts.

• Newly transplanted hair will increase in diameter and length.

• If you are planning another transplant session after your first one, wait at least eight to twelve months so that your previously transplanted hair has a chance to grow out.

• By wearing your hair short, you can expect to see your transplanted hair grow to the length of your other hair sooner than if you wear your hair longer!

• You can wear hats, scarves, or wigs while waiting for your transplanted hair to grow out to an acceptable length.

• Future transplant sessions should include the removal of the original scar from the previous session's donor site and the harvesting of an adjacent section from the donor area in order to minimize the number of scarred areas under the hair. Otherwise, a series of scars could cause a stepladder appearance in the donor areas if the hair that covers the scars is very thin.

• After the doctor places the grafts into your scalp in the direction and manner in which your hair naturally grows, you will be able to style it any way you choose once it grows, and it will look natural even when it's not combed.

• Those who have low hair density or extensive balding and little donor hair may have transplants done in what's called a *weighted* manner, in which more hair is transplanted into one area than another so that you can create a hairstyle that gives good coverage.

• Good, creative hairstyling enhances all hair transplants and should benefit women even more than men because of the many hair lengths and styling options popular for women.

Advantages of Follicular Transplants

In contrast to the larger, unnatural grafts (often called *plugs*), follicular units of one to four hairs each have numerous medical and visual advantages:

• The surgical incision at each recipient site is smaller, so healing is quicker.

• Skin surface deformity and scarring are eliminated because grafts and incisions are so small.

• Your hair will have a natural, not pluggy or doll-hair, appearance.

• Graft growth—the growth of the transplanted hairs—is superior to other types of growth.

• There are no cobblestoning scars at the recipient site. These were commonly found in surgeries involving larger grafts and incisions.

• The size of each graft is based on the natural characteristics of the patient's hair since it is determined by the naturally occurring follicular units.

• Natural scalp contour is preserved.

• Oxygen diffusion into grafts is maximized.

• Interruption of normal blood flow to the grafts is minimized in the healing phase.

• Postoperative recovery time is greatly reduced.

• Hair units may be placed very close together because they're so small.

• Large numbers of grafts may be moved per session.

• Hair is distributed in a natural pattern.

• There is great flexibility in designing recipient site areas.

Unacceptable Procedures and Tools

This list of unacceptable transplant procedures and tools describes harmful, outdated procedures that many transplant doctors are still performing and the tools used by many doctors during the procedure that are *detrimental* to good follicular transplantation. Do not agree to *any* of the methods in either category.

Unacceptable Procedures

Flap
In this barbaric procedure, a flap of skin with its tissue, hair strands, and hair follicles is shifted from the side of the head to the front hairline by cutting it on three sides, thus not separating it from its blood supply or severing it completely from the scalp.

The procedure is major surgery and is performed in a hospital. A flap is one inch wide and approximately three to seven inches long. It has to be twisted in order for the hair side of the flap to end up facing outward from the head once it's been flopped over and stitched to the balding area. A knot forms at this twist and leaves a lump. Other serious problems with this procedure are the following:

• Necrosis, or a very high chance of partial or complete death of the flap, leaving a wide, ugly scar

• Hair growing in the direction opposite from normal

• Infection

• Hair loss and extreme scarring in the donor area

• Loosened skin in the forehead hanging over the brow, giving a Frankenstein appearance

• Absence of hair behind the newly created frontal hairline

• Poor positioning of the flap

• Scarring at the stitching of the flap

• Compromised integrity of the scalp

Another kind of flap, called the *free-form flap*, is a variation on this procedure. All four sides are cut and the flap is completely removed from the donor area so that in its new position in the balding area it can be set in the direction of natural growth. Neither the flap nor the free-form flap procedure should ever be done. Although some doctors still perform this procedure on men, rarely will a female patient run into a doctor who tries to talk her into this simply because of the pattern differences in women's hair loss.

Linear or Line Grafts

In this procedure, a 3 to 4 mm linear strip of donor hair is removed from the side or back of the head. Then, instead of dividing the strip into tiny grafts, the doctor transplants the entire strip or large parts of it. Since this large graft can't be placed into tiny holes, a trench is surgically cut into the balding area and the graft is placed in the trench. As the hair grows, it looks like a line of hair so it is not cosmetically acceptable.

Round or Square Grafts

These are the original, standard, out-of-date, pluggy-looking grafts of hair. Each 3 to 5 mm graft is made with a hole-punch device and is about the size of a pencil eraser. Whether these large grafts are round or square, they are much too large and do not even remotely resemble the way hair naturally grows. When transplanted, because the grafts are so very large and therefore compromise the blood supply, the hairs in the middle of the graft often do not grow, leaving the patient with a donut effect. These large grafts are responsible for what looks like doll hair on a transplant patient's head—a pluggy look of islands of hair in an ocean of baldness, as often described. Cobblestoning scarring is very common with this procedure. Even the more recently developed smaller versions of these grafts—the minigrafts and the micrografts—can give a less than natural appearance, which is why it is recommended that transplants be comprised of only tiny grafts called *follicular units*, clusters of the one-to-four hairs that grow naturally this way in your scalp. (See the section on the follicular transplantation procedure on page 72.)

Scalp Reduction

Also known as *alopecia reduction* (AR), geleoplasty (GP), or *male pattern reduction* (MPR), scalp reductions are barbaric and disfiguring. They are performed in the doctor's office under local anesthesia. The bald part of the scalp at the top or crown of the head is literally cut away, and the edges of the nearby hair-bearing skin are sewn together, bringing the hair-bearing scalp from either side to meet in the middle. In some cases, a hideous scar results that makes the top or back of your head look like your buttocks. The scalp reduction scar sits in the middle of an area in which scalp is still often seen, so the scar looks like the "crack" between the two buttocks cheeks. Here are other problems with the scalp reduction:

• Accelerated, often permanent hair loss, more than the natural course of hair loss, which can occur within only weeks or months

• Thinning of the scalp

• An unnatural appearance because the direction of hair growth is altered

• Infection

• Hemorrhaging and hematoma (blood pooling)

• "Stretch back," in which the stretched part of the hair-bearing scalp that has been stitched together loses its tightness and stretches out partially or totally, leaving a visible scar tissue bald area created by the stretching, revealing the buttocks "crack" scar

• Suture reaction, in which the stitches in the deep layers below the skin can cause pain and swelling or in which the body can reject the sutures, causing holes in the scalp at the suture sites

Scalp reductions do not preserve hair for future use in transplants, as some physicians may try to claim, for the same wreath of permanent hair is stretched to cover a wider area in the crown, thereby thinning the permanent hair that would normally be used as donor hair for future use in transplantation.

Hair Lift

This is a more radical form of scalp reduction in which dissection or loosening of the scalp skin is done at a level below the major arteries of the scalp. To avoid damaging these blood vessels, the nerves are cut and tied. *This leaves your head permanently numb.* Unlike other scalp reductions, this form is major surgery, requiring hospitalization and general anesthesia. It leaves visible scars around the ears. Additional hair loss is often another consequence of this ill-advised procedure.

Scalp Expanders

These are silicone balloons that are inserted into pockets created between the inside of your scalp and your skull. After the incisions heal, in several weeks, the balloons are gradually inflated with a series of salt-solution injections. The head is blown up in size to two or three times its normal size. This extreme measure is done to expand scalp tissue in order to remove more tissue while creating less scalp tension prior to performing a scalp reduction. This radical procedure should *never* be done unless it's to treat trauma cases when the patient has received deep burns to the scalp.

Unacceptable Tools

Dilators

After creating the tiny slit that the transplanted hair will fit into, some doctors insert a *dilator*, a hollow steel pin that resembles a straw. They remove the dilator and then place the tiny hair graft into the dilator-widened slit. The disadvantages of using this tool include the following:

• Many doctors are unable when using dilators to control the direction in which the transplanted hair is placed and will permanently grow.

- The recipient site tissue can be damaged by the dilator.

- Recipient site pinholes have to be more widely spaced to accommodate the width of the dilators. This results in less dense coverage.

   "As grafts became smaller, some doctors had great difficulty placing the delicate grafts into the small holes or micro slits in the recipient area of the scalp," explained Dr. William Rassman. "Some doctors started using dilators. These steel pins are placed, often with some pressure, so that the doctors or technicians could locate the holes for graft placement. With time, however, many doctors have learned that these dilators were not necessary and that the grafts could be placed into the holes without them. What was required was a learning curve, something that some doctors choose *not* to learn." Dr. Rassman cautioned against relying on doctors who are unskilled in the delicate transplantation procedure. "If doctors can't do the procedure with a delicate touch, then telling the patient that dilators are the only way to do hair transplantation is like an artist telling his clients that only house-paint brushes can paint a fine Mona Lisa," he quipped.

Lasers

Some doctors have begun to use ultra- or superpulsed CO_2 lasers to create the holes at the recipient sites into which the hair grafts are inserted. Much controversy has resulted because of the following:

- Some patients have shown less hair growth in some of the laser-created sites than in scalpel-made sites. This is because the lasers currently in use compromise proper oxygenation of the transplanted graft by reducing blood flow to the area.

- Heat damage in the tissue surrounding the recipient sites can occur as the number of grafts transplanted increases.

• Hair grafts can fall out of laser-created sites because the normal skin elasticity is affected by the laser's destruction of the skin collagen and elastic fibers.

• Laser-created sites produce more scarring and more tissue death.

• Healing progresses more slowly after laser transplantation.

• Regardless of how sophisticated or precise the laser becomes it will still destroy tissue and will therefore always be inferior to a scalpel.

• Bernstein and Rassman reported in the journal *Lasers in Surgery and Medicine* (vol. 19, no. 2, 1996) that lasers were designed initially to work with an archaic transplant method — creating large, deep slits for the outdated and inferior-looking large hair plugs in procedures that are unfortunately still being performed by some doctors. In state-of-the-art follicular transplantation, however, large slits are *not* required to

> "accept the donor grafts. By identifying the patient's natural hair groupings, the implants can be pre-trimmed of the excess tissue between the groups, resulting in tiny follicular units that can be placed in very small sites, solving the problems of both recipient bulkiness and compression," they explained. "Therefore, the claim that lasers have the advantage of removing recipient tissue while creating a slit has *no* relevance in follicular transplantation."

Panel Commentary on Women as Candidates for Hair Transplantation

Dr. William Rassman

• "Since women are more desperate for hair than men, they're easier to sell. A doctor just looking to make a quick buck can make a bundle just doing women's hair transplants. Since so few women actually make good candidates for transplantation, they need to be very careful about choosing a doctor."

Dr. Robert M. Bernstein

• "Using the Densitometer, we can get a sense of how stable the hair is, we can see how much of the hair in the 'permanent zone'—the donor area—has been miniaturized. If more than 20 percent of the hair population there has been miniaturized, it's an unstable area that will continue to thin. This is the case with 90 percent of the women who have female pattern hair loss, and that does not make them acceptable candidates for hair transplantation."

• "To be a good candidate for hair transplantation, you would have to have a relatively stable donor area and good density and there would have to be a strong contrast between the back and sides and the recipient area on the front and top, similar to a male pattern of baldness."

• "Another problem for women is that they can have thin, tight scalps. A tighter scalp has less subcutaneous fat, so the incision is tighter during surgery, and that could result in hair shedding near that incision in the donor area."

• "Women with traction alopecia make excellent candidates for hair transplantation because they usually have a very good donor supply, and the hair loss is around the hairline in the front or sides."

• "Women with alopecia marginalis—a band of hair loss around the frontal edge and temples—are also good candidates for transplantation. This often looks like traction alopecia, but there is some evidence now that it's not related to traction, that it's a condition in itself, though the cause is not clear. Alopecia marginalis is found more often in black women."

• "Women who have had face-lifts and brow lifts sometimes have hair loss because of the surgical procedure itself. This affects the hairline areas only and these women make excellent transplantation candidates. We can also create eyebrows with transplanted hair from the head."

4

Extending Your Options: "Bought" Hair and Cover-Up Products

To raise new questions, new possibilities, to regard old problems from a new angle, requires creative imagination.
—Albert Einstein

Whether you're dealing with diffuse hair loss all over your head, thinning only in certain areas, the bald patches of alopecia areata, or total baldness from alopecia totalis, chemotherapy, or some other cause, one of the *best* things you can do for yourself while you are tending to the problem medically is to tend to it *cosmetically*. That means taking advantage of your many "bought" hair options. This will make you feel better by making you feel more confident about how you look.

Ignore all those well-meaning people who, in order to be polite or to make you feel like your problem isn't as bad as you think it is, tell you that "No one really notices the thinning but you," or "It's not all that bad, just ignore it," or "You're so lovely, what's a little hair loss?" If your hair loss bothers you, then it's worth addressing.

You are the only one who has to be happy about the way you look. If you're not happy, the resulting stress and anxiety will make your medical problem even worse, in a vicious circle. If you want to get better, do whatever you want to do that makes you *look* better. What a tremendous difference it will make *inside*.

"Bought" Hair

Fortunately, women have more aesthetically pleasing options than men do when it comes to wigs, hairpieces, and the like. Because many women who are suffering from hair loss keep their frontal hairlines, they're able to use wigs and hairpieces to cover thinning areas elsewhere and blend in such a way that no one would ever guess they were wearing hair that was not their own. Women whose frontal hairlines *have* been affected need not despair: Many beautiful and affordable wigs can give a very natural-looking frontal hairline, and styling options, including many types of bangs, can enhance the look even further.

Wigs, extensions, falls, and hairpieces of varying lengths and styles are so much a part of fashion these days, that plenty of women who do *not* have thinning hair are wearing them to take advantage of the different looks and lengths they can enjoy from day to day. These accessories look so natural that you would never know that they involve "bought" hair. Half the women whose hair you admire on film and television are wearing falls, extensions, and all manner of enhancements.

Visit Your Salon

Start by going to the salon that does your hair, or a new one if you'd like, and discuss your hair loss problem with the staff. Don't be embarrassed. They've seen it *all* and don't forget that they're in the business of helping people with their hair problems.

Ask about wigs, wiglets, falls, and the wide variety of locks that can be securely attached to and blended with your own hair. Many salons have these or can recommend a great place in your area where you might buy them. Your stylist can then incorporate them into your hairstyle and show you how to work with them at home. Your stylist can also recommend wigmakers, if you are interested in a custom-fitted wig, and local wig salons. Don't be shy. Ask plenty of questions and explore the options.

To Weave or Not to Weave

A weave is a way of attaching hair extensions of varying kinds to your head in a semipermanent manner. That means it stays there until the stylist removes or replaces it weeks or months later. Weaves aren't actually attached to your head but to the base of your hair where it meets your scalp. This might at first sound like a terrific idea. After all, you don't have to remove the locks at bedtime and put them in again in the morning. But it's not as great an idea as it sounds for women who have hair loss. Weaves can damage, break, and strain your existing hair, and they compromise the scalp's cleanliness and health no matter how carefully you shampoo. And the last thing a woman with hair loss needs is previously healthy hair and follicles in surrounding areas falling out or becoming damaged too.

No matter how the weaves are attached—even with gold cylinders that comprise a twenty thousand dollar "integration" process—they are a strain on your hair. Take a deep breath and say, "No thanks," and ignore the slick marketing and promises of "new and improved" techniques.

You can achieve the same effects with removable locks that won't put such strain on your hair and won't compromise your scalp's health. These can attach gently but securely and enable you to proceed with your life, even in intimate settings.

Natural or Synthetic Wigs and Pieces

Natural and synthetic wigs and locks are both good. Which type you choose will depend upon your lifestyle and on how much time you want to put into caring for and styling your "bought" hair.

You can care for natural pieces and wigs much like you care for your own hair, with shampoos, conditioners, styling products, and blow drying. Synthetic hair, however, can't be handled like natural hair—you'll use only a special shampoo, no styling products like gels, and absolutely no blow drying. The simplest wigs to care for are the synthetics—you just follow the directions for the special shampoo and conditioner, let it dry on a wig stand at room temperature, and comb it when dry. Don't go the synthetic route if you want a wig that you can wear straight as well as curly. You'll want natural hair for styling changes like that. You can, however, have a variety of synthetic wigs—straight, wavy, curly, short, long, in a wide range of colors—if you want to have styling flexibility.

Natural wigs and pieces are made from the finest human hair available (Remi Hair and Virgin European), in its natural state, which means that it has not been processed. It's strong and natural looking and the most comfortable when used for a full wig. Natural wigs and locks are more expensive than synthetic ones but last longer. Remi hair is the highest quality and the most expensive. It is soft and silky, has plenty of body, and remains tangle free.

Blends combine human hair with synthetics, are easy to care for, and have the best qualities of both types.

Wig Caps

What your wig's hair is attached to is called its *cap*. The cap is as important as the wig's hair when it comes to proper fit, comfort, and appearance. Your choice of cap will depend upon the type of hairstyle you want to have and how long you want the wig to last.

If you want to wear the wig with a part, you'll want a cap with a natural top. If you want to incorporate your own hair into the wig, you'll choose an integration cap or partial cap. If you have no hair, a full, custom-made wig with a specialized vacuum cap may be your best choice.

Capless wigs are machine made and have open construction-woven material rather than being completely closed. The top of the cap in a capless wig is closed and made of a lacy material or of a much tighter weave.

Whether the wig has a cap or is capless, you'll want the inside material to give you a cool and very light feel.

Wefted or Hand-Tied Wigs

The wig's hair is attached to the cap or interior. Wefted construction means that the cap has wefts of hair sewn into the woven material of the cap. In hand-tied construction, individual hairs are knotted by hand onto a fine nylon monofilament of polyester net base that forms the cap. Hand-tied wigs are lighter in weight, cooler, more comfortable, and natural looking.

Skin Top or French Top Wigs

Hair is hand tied into nylon mesh, and then a coating of very thin latex is applied, creating the effect of a scalp with hair growing out of it. This skin top or french top construction looks like your own skin and gives you a very natural look. Your scalp won't show through, but this wig's "scalp" will look like yours when you wear the wig parted or in other scalp-revealing styles.

Locks of Love

Locks of Love, a nonprofit organization based in Ft. Lauderdale, Florida, donates wigs to children who have lost their hair due to disease, burns, or cancer treatment. They accept donated hair. The wigs they provide are custom-made and vacuum-fit. You may want to contact them when seeking recommendations for wigmakers. See the Resource Guide for complete information.

Cover-Up Products

I am asked about cover-up products all the time. The typical question goes like this: "I see ads in magazines for what they call *cover-up products*, but if I use these, will it just look like I have a bunch of glop on my head? I know that people on television use these products all the time, but I figure that it doesn't look artificial on TV because of the lighting, camera angles, and the fact that we're not able to peer right into the actors' hair. Tell me, can someone in real life use these products successfully? Do they ever look natural?"

Well, believe it or not, they can look extremely natural. Of course it depends on the extent of your hair loss, which product you use, and how you apply it. You can use cover-up products alone or in conjunction with hair loss treatments that slow down hair loss and prompt regrowth. These cover-ups will help you feel less self-conscious while you wait for your hair loss to slow and your hair to regrow. Because women have far more styling options than men, cover-up products can be used more creatively by women. The following three products are recommended.

Toppik

Toppik consists mostly of fibers made of keratin, the same protein that is in human hair. These fibers, thousands of them, come in a nicely packaged jar. You apply Toppik by gently shaking fibers from the jar right on to the thinning areas of the scalp. The fibers attach to your existing hair—even if you have fine, wispy strands—using natural static electricity.

If you have little or moderate hair loss, Toppik will make your hair appear much fuller and natural. It comes in black, dark brown, medium brown, light brown, auburn, blond, and white. People with gray hair use the white first and then add the appropriate second color (usually dark brown or medium brown) to make the blend natural.

The 1 percent of Toppik that is not made up of organic keratin consists of approved colorant, conditioners, and glidants that keep the product flowing freely. Toppik is considered safe to use in conjunction with topical treatments like minoxidil and drugs like Propecia and other anti-androgens. You can use it after hair transplants after the recipient sites have healed. It's particularly useful after transplants while you're waiting for your new hair to grow out.

It washes out easily and won't damage your hair or scalp, yet it doesn't come off easily during daily wear, not even if it's windy or rainy. It won't brush out, so you can comb your hair during the day and even run your fingers through it without worrying that it will come out. It will come out, however, if you swim underwater. Because it doesn't stain or streak, you don't have to worry if it gets on your clothes while you're shaking it on — just brush it right off.

Couvre Masking Lotion

Couvre was the first camouflage product for hair loss. It gained widespread usage among theatre makeup artists. This is a scalp coloring that you apply with a special sponge applicator that comes with the product. Couvre masks hair loss underneath some hair, which means that you can't put it on bald spots unless there's a fair amount of hair covering those areas. It's great for thinning areas, no matter how large or small. It eliminates the contrast between your scalp and your hair and also thickens the base of the hairs so that they appear much thicker overall. You can't use it on your hairline edges, but you can use it all over the scalp under existing moderately thinning hair, and it will look natural. It only comes off when you shampoo it out. It won't come off in the rain, and you can even swim with it and it won't run or smear.

It can be applied to either damp or dry hair and scalp and takes only about a minute to fully set. It doesn't clog pores or interfere with hair growth.

Couvre is much like a colored moisturizer. Its main ingredients are sesame oil, often used as a natural moisturizer base in skin care products, and iron oxides, which are naturally derived colorants approved for use around the face and even the eyes. You can use it with minoxidil or any other topical treatment— just put the Couvre on last after your topical treatment has been completely absorbed. At night, you can apply minoxidil right over the Couvre, although the alcohol in the minoxidil solution will remove some of the Couvre and you'll have to do a touch-up. Couvre comes in eight colors—black, dark brown, medium brown, light brown, auburn, blond, gray, and white-gray.

Fullmore Colored Hair Thickener

This new product is like a combination of Toppik and Couvre in a spray form that delivers tiny colored fibers to your thinning hair and scalp but with none of the messy, hard-to-control problems of the previous generation of spray cover-up products. It is made of the same keratin fibers as Toppik and comes in the same colors.

5

In the Works: Treatments in Research

Ingenuity plus courage plus work equals miracles.
—Bob Richards

I wish that I could tell you that cures are just around the corner, but I can't. And that's not because research isn't progressing. Nor is it because hair loss conditions are so mysterious that it could take decades before anyone gets a handle on possible cures. The reason is insidious: *Cures may very well be possible, but it's not in a pharmaceutical company's best financial interest to provide a cure, only to provide treatments that will continue to rake in the dollars day after day, month after month, year after year.*

Pharmaceutical companies are first and foremost *businesses*. They are *for profit*. And they have to answer to shareholders who expect a return on their investment. Period.

What a wonderful world it would be if all pharmaceutical companies were nonprofit businesses, for whom the incentive to develop products was completely altruistic and had nothing to do with an endless stream of profit. But, at least in the foreseeable future, we're stuck with our current system.

I once heard a rather eye-opening story about an inventor and businessman who was remembering a lesson his electronics instructor taught him in his student days. It was about a concept called *planned obsolescence.* Simply put, the concept refers to the notion that products must be designed so that they will become obsolete, so that they will wear out (and sooner, rather than later), and so that consumers will have to purchase new ones on a fairly regular basis. Certainly, the instructor said, we could create a lightbulb that would never burn out, and we could create a toaster that would last for thirty years, but that would put the lightbulb and toaster companies out of business very quickly.

The goal, in this class, was simply to build a great product, not to build one that would last forever. If you did *that,* you failed the class. Why? Because that would be the *last* thing in the world a company would want from one of its inventors, engineers, or other specialists.

Drugs and other treatment options in the medical world, which is as profit oriented as any other for profit business, are created entirely with profit in mind. There is, perhaps, one exception to this rule, and that is the treatment of contagious disease. Cures and vaccines pop up quickly for the most complex, devastating, highly contagious maladies of the world. The reason is that a contagious disease that's extremely debilitating or fatal can have an overwhelming negative *economic* impact on an entire local, regional, national, or even international area and quite quickly. So, even in the case of deadly, contagious diseases, economics plays a key role.

Doctors, researchers, and even those working in the pharmaceutical industry are well aware of the effect of economics on medicine. Routinely, those nearing possible cures are discredited or ignored. When Columbia University researcher and geneticist Angela Christiano, Ph.D., discovered the first gene linked to hair loss, she experienced the strong effect of economics. As writer John Sedgwick reported in the May 1999 issue of GQ magazine in an investigative article about Christiano's work and the politics and economics of the pharmaceutical industry, "It may well be that the drug companies are acting disdainfully of Christiano for the simple reason that they are far less interested in finding a one-shot baldness cure than in developing a continuing treatment . . . that generates lucrative repeat business. The University of Miami's [Dr.] Marty Sawaya suspects as much: "I've been told by industry people, 'We don't want to cure a disease, we just want to treat it so we will continue to have people to buy our stuff.'" Then she adds, "But if you ask them about it directly, they'll definitely deny it."

As Sedgwick reminds us, worldwide there are fewer than one hundred hair research specialists, so it's clear that individual scientists as well as drug companies aren't exactly falling over each other in a mad dash to bring hair loss sufferers any real relief anytime soon. Dr. Angela Christiano is a rarity in that she is an intensely committed lone scientist hunkered down in the lab with very little funding, personally driven to find answers while ignoring the political and economic swirl around her.

After a bout with alopecia areata, Dr. Christiano changed the focus of her dermatological research to hair, specifically to finding genes responsible for hair loss. In October 1997, in her modest lab at Columbia, funded by a tiny grant from the Alopecia Areata Foundation, Christiano found the very first gene linked to hair loss. It was a monumental event in genetic science and only took her seventeen months. Dubbed "the hairless gene," this particular gene caused a very rare, inherited kind of alopecia that involved complete hairlessness of the entire body from birth in a Pakistani family. It is so significant because it opens the door to the discovery of other hair loss genes.

Her findings were published in January 1998 in the journal *Science*. The article received enormous worldwide publicity. At age thirty-three, Christiano has published more than one hundred articles in major scientific journals.

As Christiano notes, genetic research in hair is about fifty years behind the rest of genetics. A gene could have been discovered years ago had anybody bothered to look for it as diligently and creatively as Christiano did.

New Treatments in Research

Here is a list of some of the most promising new preventions and treatments currently in research or development. Some may be available very soon, others are within five years of reaching the market, some are currently available outside the country and may soon be heading for the U.S. market, and others are in early or intermediate stages of research and development.

Gene Therapy

After discovering the "hairless gene," Dr. Christiano applied the principles of "the nude gene," which causes a certain kind of hair loss in mice, to people. She continues her research, with the goal of finding the genes linked to alopecia areata, androgenetic alopecia (male and female pattern baldness), and other hair loss disorders.

A San Diego biotech company, AntiCancer, Inc., has developed a way to deliver a gene's DNA coding directly to hair follicles. Once genes for hair loss are identified, this company's gene delivery method may be employed.

Cloning

By cloning just one of your hairs, scientists will be able to make as many hairs as you need to completely fill in all of your thinning areas during transplant procedures. Dr. Colin Jahoda of the University of Durham, in England, is the world's leading authority on hair cloning (also called *hair culturing*) technology and its potential for treating hair loss. Research in this area is also ongoing at the University of Washington in Seattle and elsewhere. Scientists have already been able to grow hair in the lab, and Dr. Jahoda has grown a cloned hair on his arm.

PTH

Dr. Michael Holick of Boston University Medical School and researchers in Berlin have shown that hair follicles can return to their growing phase when PTHrP, a chemical in the body that causes hair follicles to go into a resting cycle (and hair to enter its shedding cycle), is blocked. The blocking agent is called PTH, and studies in mice show that scientists may have found the equivalent of the switch that turns hair growth back on. Human studies are scheduled for testing PTH.

Buserelin

Researchers in Italy are studying the effects of the drug Buserelin in the treatment of women with excess body and facial hair (hirsutism). Because the same hormonal actions that cause hirsutism are also responsible for most hormone-triggered female pattern baldness, Buserelin may become a future treatment for hair loss in women. The drug reduces the secretion of androgens by ovaries that have ovarian cysts. No significant side effects have been observed.

Other 5-Alpha Reductase Inhibitors

Proscar (5 mg finasteride) inhibits the enzyme 5-alpha reductase, thereby inhibiting DHT production by 70 percent. Propecia

(1 mg finasteride) inhibits DHT production by 60 percent. Merck, the pharmaceutical company that makes those drugs, is working on more ways to inhibit this enzyme which converts testosterone into hair follicle–killing DHT. Drugs that will work faster than finasteride and that can safely inhibit DHT production up to 98 percent are in the research and development phase.

Aromatase

Aromatase is an enzyme in the body that blocks or deactivates DHT's effect on hair follicles. Researchers are studying it to determine its use as a hair loss prevention and treatment.

Cyoctol

Cyoctol, a new drug in development at Upjohn, the pharmaceutical company that makes Rogaine (minoxidil), blocks the effects of testosterone on hair follicles, slowing down hair loss and triggering regrowth. Cyoctol is used as a topical lotion applied to the scalp. It is still in the human-testing phase. Preliminary results show that 92 percent of the men in a one-year test showed some slowing of hair loss and some hair regrowth. Drugs like this that are initially developed for men can often be used by women under certain circumstances.

RU 58841

One of the most promising hair loss drugs in development is caught in the middle of a corporate tug-of-war, and rumors abound that it's being suppressed because it works *too well* and would be a major threat to the current prominent hair loss drugs on the market today. This suppression is rumored to be at the hands of a competitor who may have found a way to own or license the drug. This topical drug, RU 58841, is an androgen-receptor blocker. It inhibits the effects of testosterone and DHT on hair follicles.

"It's a good topical agent. I did some of the work on it a few years ago," says one of the country's leading hair loss physicians and researchers, Dr. Marty Sawaya, who is quoted frequently in this book as part of our expert panel. "It's a political internal problem. The company decided not to go forward with it. There are companies trying to license it from them and then develop it."

Will it be developed, or will it be kept off the market by a competitor who licenses it? Time will tell, but as of this writing, RU 58841 is still in limbo and nowhere near being readied for the marketplace.

Nitroxide (TEMPOL)

The topical compound nitroxide radical TEMPOL is currently being studied by the Radiation Oncology Branch of the National Cancer Institute for its ability to prevent radiation-induced baldness during the treatment of cancer and other conditions. Initial studies look promising.

Hair Growth Gene

In October, 1999, gene therapists at the Weill Medical College of Cornell University reported in the *Journal of Clinical Investigation* that they had successfully injected a gene into mice that forces resting hair follicles into the growing phase. The gene, nicknamed "Sonic Hedgehog," a hereditary factor essential for development, was carried into the mice by a virus used simply as a transportation mechanism. The research has not been tried on humans, and researchers still need to contend with the fact that overactivity of the Sonic Hedgehog gene is a cause of basal cell carcinoma, which is a common yet treatable skin cancer.

Appendix A
Prescription Drugs That Can Cause Hair Loss

Many commonly prescribed prescription drugs can cause temporary hair loss, trigger the onset of female (and male) pattern baldness, and even cause permanent hair loss. The drugs in this appendix do *not* include those used in chemotherapy and radiation for the treatment of cancer.

Your doctor may not mention hair loss as a side effect of some drugs, so don't forget to do your own research and read the drug manufacturer's complete warnings regarding the drug. Your pharmacist can provide you with this information even before you fill a prescription. Many pill and medication guidebooks (sold in bookstores and pharmacies) are excellent sources of complete information on prescription drugs.

If your doctor prescribes any of the following drugs, ask if one that does *not* have hair loss as a possible side effect can be substituted. The brand names of the drugs are listed first, followed by the drug's generic name in parentheses. The drugs are listed by category, according to the conditions they treat. In some categories, individual drugs are not listed, and you will want to discuss the possibility of hair loss as a side effect of using *any* of the drugs that treat that particular condition, since many of them *do* contribute to hair loss.

Acne

All drugs derived from vitamin A as treatments for acne or other conditions, including

- Accutane (isotretinoin)

Blood

Anticoagulants (blood thinners), including

- Panwarfin
- Sofarin   (warfarin sodium)
- Coumadin
- Heparin injections

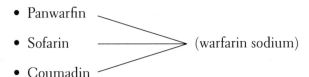

Cholesterol

Cholesterol-lowering drugs, including

- Atronid-S (clofibrate)
- Lopid (gemfibrozil)

Convulsions, Epilepsy

Anticonvulsants, including

- Tridone (trimethadione)

Depression

Antidepression drugs, including

- Prozac (fluoxetine hydrochloride)
- Zoloft (sertraline hydrochloride)
- Paxil (paroxetine)
- Anafranil (clomipramine)
- Janimine
- Tofranil — (imipramine)
- Tofranil PM
- Adapin
- Sinequan — (doxepin)
- Surmontil (trimipramine)
- Pamelor
- Ventyl — (nortriptyline)
- Elavin
- Endep — (amitriptyline)
- Norpramin
- Pertofrane — (desipramine)
- Vivactil (protriptyline hydrochloride)
- Asendin (amoxapine)
- Haldol (haloperidol)

Fungus

Antifungals

Glaucoma

The beta-blocker drugs, including

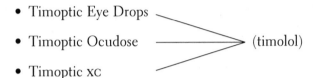

- Timoptic Eye Drops
- Timoptic Ocudose   (timolol)
- Timoptic XC

Gout

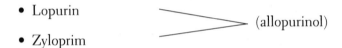

- Lopurin
- Zyloprim   (allopurinol)

Heart Conditions

Many drugs prescribed for the heart, including those known as the beta blockers, which are also used to treat high blood pressure, including

- Tenormin (atenolol)
- Lopressor (metoprolol)
- Corgard (nadolol)
- Inderal and Inderal LA (propanolol)
- Blocadren (timolol)

High Blood Pressure

See list of beta blockers under Heart Conditions.

Hormonal Conditions

All hormone-containing drugs and drugs prescribed for hormone-related, reproductive, male-specific, and female-specific conditions and situations, including

• Birth control pills (even though some with a higher progesterone content and lower androgenic effect are used to treat hair loss)

• Hormone replacement therapy (HRT) for women (estrogen and progesterone, even though some combinations are used to treat hair loss)

• Male androgenic hormones and all forms of testosterone

• Anabolic steroids

• Prednisone and other steroids

Inflammation

Many anti-inflammatory drugs, including those prescribed for localized pain, swelling, and injury

• Arthritis drugs

• Nonsteroidal anti-inflammatory drugs (NSAIDs), including

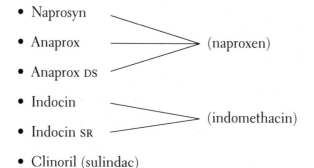

     • Naprosyn

     • Anaprox   (naproxen)

     • Anaprox DS

     • Indocin

     • Indocin SR   (indomethacin)

     • Clinoril (sulindac)

Anti-inflammatory drugs also used as chemotherapy drugs, including

- Methotrexate (MTX)
- Rheumatex 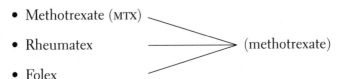 (methotrexate)
- Folex

Overweight

Amphetamines

Parkinson's Disease

- Levadopa/L-dopa (dopar, laradopa)

Thyroid Disorders

Many of the drugs used to treat the thyroid

Ulcer

Many of the drugs used to treat indigestion, stomach difficulties, and ulcers, in over-the-counter dosages and prescription dosages, including

- Tagamet (cimetidine)
- Zantac (ranitidine)
- Pepcid (famotidine)

Appendix B
The Savin Female
Hair Loss Scale

There are two widely known female hair loss density scales used by most hair loss specialists: the Ludwig Scale and the Savin Scale (see following page). For all intents and purposes, they are identical except that the Savin Scale also measures overall thinning. For that reason, I decided to include the Savin Scale and not the perhaps more well-known Ludwig Scale in this book.

As you will see in these illustrations, eight crown density images reflect a range from *no hair loss* to *severe hair loss*. Density 8 is rarely seen in clinical practice. One example of frontal anterior recession is also illustrated (again, it's not too common), and one example of general diffuse thinning, lateral view, is shown.

Savin Female Hair Loss Scale

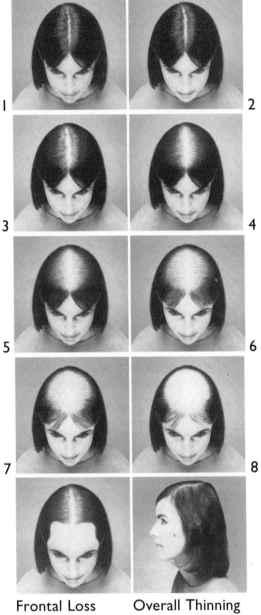

Frontal Loss   Overall Thinning

The Savin Scale courtesy of Pharmacia & Upjohn Company

Appendix C
Resource Guide

Recommended Reading

Books on Hair Loss

The Bald Truth, by Spencer David Kobren (Pocket, 1998).

Skin Deep: An A–Z of Skin Disorders, Treatments, and Health, by Carol A. Turkington, Jeffrey S. Dover (Facts on File, 1996).

The Life of the Skin, by Arthur K. Balin, Loretta Pratt Balin, Marietta Whittlesey (Bantam Doubleday Dell, 1997).

Alopecia Areata: Understanding and Coping with Hair Loss, by Wendy Thompson and Jerry Shapiro (Johns Hopkins University Press, 1996).

The Big Fall: Living with Hair Loss, by Sheila Jacobs (Next Century Books, 1992).

Books Helpful for Women's Health

Woman Heal Thyself, by Jeanne Elizabeth Blum (Charles E. Tuttle, 1995).

The Harvard Guide to Women's Health, by Karen J. Carlson, M.D., Stephanie A. Eisenstat, M.D., and Terra Ziporyn, Ph.D. (Harvard University Press, 1995).

Women's Bodies, Women's Wisdom (revised edition), by Christiane Northrup, M.D. (Bantam Books, 1998).

Voices of Truth: Conversations with Scientists, Thinkers & Healers, by Nina L. Diamond (Lotus Press, 2000).

Purify Your Body: Natural Remedies for Detoxing from 50 Everyday Situations, by Nina L. Diamond (Crown/Three Rivers Press, 1997).

Reclaiming Our Health, by John Robbins (H. J. Kramer, 1996).

Ageless Body, Timeless Mind, by Deepak Chopra, M.D. (Harmony Books, 1993).

Encyclopedia of Natural Medicine, by Joe Pizzorno, N.D., and Michael Murray, N.D. (Prima Publishing, 1991).

Total Wellness, by Joe Pizzorno, N.D. (Prima Publishing, 1996).

The Zone, by Barry Sears, Ph.D. (Regan Books, 1995).

The Essential Guide to Vitamins and Minerals, by Elizabeth Somer (HarperCollins, 1995).

Health and Healing (revised edition), by Andrew Weill, M.D. (Houghton Mifflin, 1995).

Natural Health, Natural Medicine (revised edition), by Andrew Weill, M.D. (Houghton Mifflin, 1995).

Spontaneous Healing, by Andrew Weill, M.D. (Knopf, 1995).

In the House of the Moon, by Jason Elias, Katherine Ketchum (Warner Books, 1995).

Herbal Healing for Women, by Rosemary Gladstar (Simon & Schuster, 1993).

Red Moon Passage, by Bonnie J. Horrigan (Harmony Books, 1996).

What Every Woman Needs to Know About Estrogen, by Karen Anne Hutchinson, M.D. (Plume, 1997).

Menopause Without Medicine (3d edition), by Linda Ojeda, Ph.D. (Hunter House, 1995).

What Your Doctor May Not Tell You About Menopause, by John R. Lee, M.D., Virginia Hopkins (Warner Books, 1996).

What Your Doctor May Not Tell You About Pre-Menopause, by John R. Lee, M.D., Virginia Hopkins, Jesse Hanley (Warner Books, 1999).

Inner Peace, Outer Beauty, by Michelle Dominique Leigh (Citadel Press, 1995).

Publications

Natural Health
    P.O. Box 7440
    Red Oak, IA 51591
    (800) 526-8440
    The country's best magazine about natural health; bimonthly

HerbalGram, Journal of the American Botanical Council and the Herbal Research Foundation
   (512) 331-8868
   Thorough and authoritative publication; call the Botanical Council bookstore at (800) 373-7105

Dermatologic Surgery
   930 North Meacham Road
   Schaumburg, IL 60173
   Medical journal

International Journal of Aesthetic and Restorative Surgery
   c/o George Faber, M.D., Secretary
   200 West Esplanade Avenue, #102
   Kenner, LA 70065
   (504) 471-3130
   Medical journal

Websites

These three websites offer the most comprehensive information regarding hair loss. They can also link you to scores of other pertinent sites.

- www.thebaldtruth.org (the author's website)

- www.keratin.com

- www.hairtoday.com

Organizations

The following list does not include any of the medical associations among whose members are doctors who perform hair transplantation surgery or any of the trade associations in the hair loss "industry." This omission is completely intentional because those associations will recommend members who may still be performing outdated procedures that can be harmful and leave the patient with aesthetically unacceptable results.

For a list of recommended physicians who specialize in hair loss and also those who perform follicular transplantation, see those sections in this Resource Guide.

The organizations listed here can provide you with information for your hair loss research, prevention, and treatment efforts.

National Institutes of Health (NIH)
    Office of Alternative Medicine (OAM)
    6120 Executive Blvd., #450
    Rockville, MD 20892
    (301) 402-2466

The NIH is a government agency that funds and coordinates research and clinical studies in all areas of health and medicine, including alternative or natural medicine. The OAM can give you information regarding its department and can also refer you to other departments for pharmaceutical studies and other pertinent research.

National Alopecia Areata Foundation
    P.O. Box 150760
    San Rafael, CA 94915
    (415) 456-4274

National Women's Health Resource Center
    2440 M Street N.W., Suite 325
    Washington, DC 10037
    (202) 293-6045

National Black Women's Health Project
    1237 Ralph Abernathy Blvd. S.W.
    Atlanta, GA 30310
    (800) 275-2947

National Latina Health Organization
    P.O. Box 7567
    Oakland, CA 94601
    (510) 534-1362

National Women's Health Network
    514 10th Street N.W.
    Washington, DC 20004
    (202) 347-1140

Women to Women/Christiane Northrup, M.D.
    One Pleasant Street
    Yarmouth, ME 04096
    (207) 846-6163

Womens International Pharmacy
    (800) 279-5708
    Prescription drugs and natural medicines can be ordered by
your doctor from this pharmacy.

American Asssociation of Naturopathic Physicians
    2366 Eastlake Ave. East
    Suite 322
    Seattle, WA 98102
    (206) 328-8510

American Herbalists Guild
    Box 1683
    Soquel, CA 95073
    (408) 464-2441

Herb Research Foundation
   1007 Pearl Street, #200
   Boulder, CO 80302
   (303) 440-2265

American Holistic Medical Association
   4101 Lake Boone Trail, #201
   Raleigh, NC 27607
   (919) 787-5146

Association of Natural Medicine Pharmacists
   (707) 887-1351
   This organization provides pharmacists with up-to-date scientific information on natural medicines.

American Cancer Society
   1599 Clifton Road N.E.
   Atlanta, GA 30329
   (404) 320-3333

Skin Cancer Foundation
   245 Fifth Avenue, #1403
   New York, NY 10016
   (212) 725-5176

American Hemochromatosis Society (AHS)
   777 East Atlantic Avenue, #Z-363
   Delray Beach, FL 33483
   www.americanhs.org
   Hemochromatosis is an iron overload condition.

Hemochromatosis Research Foundation
   P.O. Box 8569
   Albany, NY 12208
   (518) 489-0972

Scleroderma Research Foundation
   Pueblo Medical Commons
   2320 Bath St., #307
   Santa Barbara, CA 93105
   (805) 563-1164
   (800) 441-CURE

National Organization for Rare Disorders
   P.O. Box 8923
   New Fairfield, CT 06812
   (203) 746-6518
   (800) 999-6673

Trichotillomania Learning Center
   1215 Mission St., #2
   Santa Cruz, CA 95060
   (408) 457-1004
   Trichotillomania is a hair-pulling disorder.

Polycystic Ovarian Syndrome Association
   P.O. Box 7007
   Rosemont, IL 60018
   www.pcosupport.org

Lupus Foundation of America
   1300 Piccard Drive, #200
   Rockville, MD 20850
   (301) 670-9292
   (800) 558-0121

American Lupus Society
   3914 Del Amo Blvd., #922
   Torrance, GA 90503
   (213) 542-8891
   (800) 331-9802

National Psoriasis Foundation/International Federation of
      Psoriasis Foundations
   6600 S.W. 92nd, #300
   Portland, OR 97223
   (503) 244-7404

Scleroderma Foundation
   89 Newbury Street, #201
   Danvers, MA 01923
   (978) 750-4499
   (800) 422-1113

Hair Loss Researchers

Research breakthroughs often come from the study of a particular person or a group of people with hair loss. As you read in Chapter Five, Dr. Angela Christiano discovered the very first gene linked to hair loss when she heard about a family in Pakistan who had a rare, inherited form of hairlessness, and she arranged to study them.

Researchers may also be able to provide you with information regarding clinical studies of treatments you may be eligible to participate in. You in turn may be of help to researchers by providing them with accounts of your experiences with certain hair loss treatments and preventions.

Three leading researchers whose work is detailed in this book may be contacted at their offices listed here:

Angela M. Christiano, Ph.D.
Columbia University College of Physicians and Surgeons
630 West 168th Street, VC-1526
New York, NY 10032
(212) 305-9565
amc65@columbia.edu

Dr. Colin Jahoda
Professor, Department of Biological Sciences
Durham University
Stockton Road
Durham DH1 3LY
England
Phone: 0191-374-3018

Dr. Marty E. Sawaya, M.D.
Aratec
P.O. Box 7
Ocala, FL 34478
(352) 867-7611

Hair Loss Physicians

The physicians on this list specialize in the treatment of hair loss in both men and women, a subspecialty in dermatology. Each of these physicians participates in research but is also in private practice and sees patients on a regular basis.

Although this list is brief, these physicians are considered by their peers to be among the best in the country in the diagnosis and treatment of hair loss problems, and they can recommend physicians of equal caliber in your area. They may also be available to consult with the physicians you are currently seeing. Because these physicians are active in ongoing research, they can also consult with you regarding treatments in development and patient participation in clinical trials for new treatments.

This list is presented in alphabetical order.

Marty E. Sawaya, M.D., Ph.D.
Aratec
P.O. Box 7
Ocala, FL 34478
(352) 867-7611

• Is a dermatologist (board certified)

• Is Principal Investigator of Clinical Research at ARATEC (Alopecia Research and Associated Technologists), Ocala, Florida

• Is Adjunct Professor of Biochemistry and Molecular Biology at the University of Miami School of Medicine, where she continues her basic scientific research

• Received doctor of medicine degree from the University of Miami School of Medicine, 1983

• Received Ph.D. from the University of Miami, 1986

• Did research postdoctoral training at the University of Miami, 1987–1988

• Was resident in dermatology at SUNY (State University of New York), Brooklyn, and the University of Florida

• Research focused in the field of steroid biochemistry as it relates to skin diseases, especially hair diseases such as androgenetic alopecia and alopecia areata

• Received research grant from the NIH (National Institutes of Health), 1992–1997

- Received multiple research grants from the National Alopecia Areata Foundation, 1989–1995

- Current clinical research also focused on skin cancers; current work integrates with hair diseases in the study of the hair follicle cycle and regulation of the cell death mechanisms

- Recently received a Merck Education Research Grant and formed research collaborations with Merck-Frosst, Canada, in the study of dermatological diseases

- Current clinical research includes ongoing clinical trials for Glaxo-Wellcome for a new oral drug for treatment of men with androgenetic alopecia (male pattern baldness); for Bristol Myers-Squibb for a new topical cream to arrest hair growth for women with facial hair; for Pharmacia and Upjohn for 5 percent minoxidil for women with hair loss; for Bristol Myers-Squibb for a new topical cream, eflornithine hydrocloride, for men with pseudofolliculitis; and for Neutrogena Co. for a new topical lotion for treating men's and women's hair loss

- Consults with various pharmaceutical companies for product research and development as related to dermatology, with emphasis on hair and other skin diseases; has published two dozen research papers, twelve book chapters, thirty-six abstracts; is co-editor of a book in preparation for publication

- Is available for private practice consultation

Kenneth J. Washenik, M.D., Ph.D.
Dermatopharmacology Unit/Department of Dermatology
NYU Medical Center
560 First Avenue, #H-158
New York, NY 10016
(212) 263-5244

• Is a dermatologist (board certified, American Board of Dermatology, Fellow of the American Academy of Dermatology)

• Is Director of Dermatopharmacology Unit, NYU Medical Center, New York, New York, 1996, present, and Assistant Professor, Department of Dermatology

• Has dermatology clinical practice, New York, New York, 1994–present

• Was Chief of Dermatology, Department of Medicine, Brooklyn Hospital Center, Brooklyn, New York, 1995–1997

• Received bachelor of science in biology from the Philadelphia College of Pharmacy and Science (PCPS), 1981

• Received doctor of medicine degree and Ph.D. from Baylor College of Medicine, Houston, Texas, 1990

• Did internship at St. Joseph Hospital, Houston, Texas, 1990–1991

• Did residency in dermatology at New York University Medical Center, New York, New York, 1991–1994

• Received Dermatopharmacology Fellowship at NYU Medical Center, 1994–1995

• Was Staff Dermatologist, Bronx-Lebanon Hospital, New York, New York, 1994–1996; Attending Physician in Dermatology, New York Veterans Affairs Medical Center, New York, New York, 1995–1996

• Has received many academic and research awards; has presented his research at medical and clinical conferences across the country

• Specialties include the treatment of androgenetic alopecia and other hair loss

Hair Transplantation Physicians

The physicians listed here perform state-of-the-art follicular transplantation. They are recognized by their peers as leaders in the field, not only for their medical expertise and integrity, but also for their active role in educating their fellow physicians also (as well as patients) in the most recent and welcome innovations for safe and effective hair transplantation surgery. These physicians also conduct research, publish in respected medical journals, present research findings and techniques at medical conferences, and are vocal advocates for continued change in the field.

Because an excellent physician skilled at follicular transplantation may not be located in your city or even your state, you may want to keep in mind that many patients travel for their transplantation procedures, which are performed in one day at the doctor's medical office. The physicians on this list may also be able to recommend equally skilled physicians in your area.

This guide is presented in alphabetical order.

Michael Beehner, M.D.
10 Railroad Place, #102
Saratoga Springs, NY 12866
(518) 581-1872

• Is a surgeon

• Is family medicine board certified by the American Board of Family Practice

• Is Associate Clinical Professor of Medicine at Albany Medical Center, Albany, New York

• Was 1995 recipient of the Outstanding Achievement Award presented by the American Academy of Facial Plastic and Reconstructive Surgery

- Graduated from Loyola University, 1967

- Received doctor of medicine degree from the University of Illinois Medical School, 1971

- Interned in family practice at Wesley Medical Center in Wichita, Kansas, 1971–1972

- Did residency in general surgery at St. Francis Medical Center in Wichita, Kansas, 1974–1975

- Did residency in family practice at the University of Wisconsin, 1975–1977

- Was with the U.S. Public Health Service's National Health Service Corps., stationed in West Winfield, New York, 1972–1974, between his internship and his first residency

- Has served as president of the medical staff at Moses-Ludinton Hospital in Ticonderoga, New York, and as president of the Essex County Medical Society

- Is active in a number of professional societies

- Is active in hair-transplant surgery research and clinical presentations

- Publication credits include "The Frontal Forelock Concept in Hair Replacement Surgery" in the *American Journal of Cosmetic Surgery* (1997) and "A Frontal Forelock/Central Density Framework for Hair Transplantation" in *Dermatologic Surgery Journal* (1997); his work has also appeared in *International Hair Transplant Forum*

- Has lectured and performed live surgery at the Annual Live Surgery Workshop and presented lectures at the annual meeting of the International Society of Hair Replacement Surgery

Robert M. Bernstein, M.D.
2150 Center Avenue
Fort Lee, NJ 07024
(201) 585-1115

• Is a dermatologist (board certified in dermatology, Fellow of the American Academy of Dermatology)

• Is Assistant Clinical Professor of Dermatology at the College of Physicians and Surgeons of Columbia University, New York, New York

• Is Associate in the Dermatology Service, Columbia-Presbyterian Medical Center, New York, New York, where he teaches dermatologic and laser surgery and hair transplantation.

• Graduated cum laude from Tulane University; was named Tulane scholar

• Was awarded doctor of medicine degree by the University of Medicine and Dentistry of New Jersey; was recipient of the Dr. Jacob Bleiberg Award for Excellence in Dermatology

• Is Chief Resident, Dermatology, Albert Einstein College of Medicine, New York, New York

• First introduced the technique of follicular transplantation in the *International Journal of Aesthetic and Restorative Surgery* and at the International Society of Hair Restoration Surgery

• Was named "Surgeon of the Month," *Hair Transplant Forum International*

• Has recently published articles: "Follicular Transplantation: Patient Evaluation and Surgical Planning" and "The Aesthetics of Follicular Transplantation"

• Is active in clinical research, teaching, and medical society lectures

Roy Jones, M.D.
  1840 Mesquite Avenue, Suite D
  Lake Havasu City, AZ 86403
  (520) 855-3077

• Is a surgeon (board certified by the American Board of Surgery)

• Graduated from Wichita State University, 1970

• Received doctor of medicine degree from the University of Kansas School of Medicine, 1974

• Combined rotating internship and general surgery residency at the University of Kansas, Wichita, 1974–1979

• Served as Chief of Surgery at Wurtsmith Air Force Base Hospital, Michigan

• Served as Vice Chairman of the Nevada State Emergency Medical System's Trauma Task Force

• Served on the American College of Surgeons' Committee on Trauma, and has been an advanced trauma life-support instructor

• Is active in professional societies, encouraging the advancement of hair transplantation surgery

Robert Blaine Lehr, M.D.
  5701 N. Portland, #310
  Oklahoma City, OK 73112
  (405) 951-4970

• Is a dermatologist (board certified by the American Board of Dermatology)

• Is an associate of Dr. O'Tar Norwood, creator of the Norwood Scale for measuring male pattern baldness

• Graduated from the University of Oklahoma, 1986, with honors

• Received doctor of medicine degree from the University of Oklahoma College of Medicine, 1990; received numerous awards there, including the Tom Lowry Award for ranking first in the class after his first year and the Mark R. Everett Award for most promising second-year student

• Did internship at Baptist Medical Center, Oklahoma City, 1990–1991

• Did residency in dermatology at the University of Oklahoma, 1992–1995

• Publishes frequently in *Hair Transplant Forum Journal* and is a member of a number of professional societies

Bobby L. Limmer, M.D.
    14615 San Pedro Ave., Suite 210
    One Medical Park
    San Antonio, TX 78232
    (210) 496-9929

• Is a dermatologist (board certified by the American Board of Dermatology)

• Introduced the use of the microscope into the hair transplantation procedure (see Chapter Three) and has been at the forefront of transplantation innovations, giving more than thirty presentations at prestigious medical conferences and publishing more than a dozen articles in leading medical journals, including *Dermatologic Surgery, Advances in Dermatology, Dermatologic Surgery and Oncology,* and *Hair Transplant Forum International*

• Graduated magna cum laude from Texas A&M University, 1964

• Received doctor of medicine degree from the University of Texas, Galveston, 1968

• Did internship at Fitzsimons General Hospital, Denver, 1968–1969

• Did residency in dermatology at Brooke Army Medical Center, San Antonio, Texas, 1969–1972

• Served in the U.S. Army Medical Corps, 1966–1974, receiving a U.S. Army Commendation medal

• Has received many academic appointments and fellowships and has been a clinical professor at the University of Texas Health Center, San Antonio

• Is active in professional societies and has held a number of offices, including president of the San Antonio Dermatologic Society and chairman of the board of directors of the American College of Cryosurgery

• Received the Platinum Follicle Award, 1996, presented annually to one individual by the International Society of Hair Restoration Surgery for the most important basic research in hair anatomy and physiology in the world

Robert E. McClellan, M.D.
    9911 West Pico Blvd.
    Los Angeles, CA 90035
    (310) 553-9113

• Is a surgeon (board certified by the American Board of Surgery)

• Received doctor of medicine degree from the University of Utah School of Medicine, 1975

• Did internship in surgery at Providence Hospital in Southfield, Michigan

• Was a medical doctor and regimental surgeon for the U.S. Navy, stationed in Okinawa, Japan, and Brunswick, Maine, 1976–1978

• Did residency in general surgery at Berkshire Medical Center, Pittsfield, Massachusetts

• Was instructor in general surgery at the University of Massachusetts Medical School

• Had general surgery practice in Utah and Wyoming, 1982–1988; practice devoted full-time to hair transplantation since then

O'Tar Norwood, M.D.
    5710 N. Portland, #310
    Oklahoma City, OK 73112
    (405) 951-4970

• Is a dermatologist (board certified by the American Board of Dermatology)

• Is Associate Clinical Professor of Dermatology, University of Oklahoma Health Sciences Center

• Set the standard for classifying degrees of male pattern baldness with the Norwood Scale

• Wrote "Male Pattern Baldness Classification Incidence," 1975, a classic that remains the standard today and is used by all hair-transplant surgeons and physicians from all over the world when dealing with men's hair loss

• Has published more than thirty articles

• Is a teacher and lecturer

• Is co-founder of the International Society for Hair Restoration Surgery

• Is founder, editor, and publisher of the bimonthly publication *Hair Transplant Forum International*

• Graduated from the University of Arkansas, 1953

• Received doctor of medicine degree from the University of Arkansas Medical School, 1957

• Did internship at the U.S. Navy Hospital in Oakland, California

• Did residency in dermatology at the University of Oklahoma, 1961–1964

• Is active in numerous professional societies and has held many offices, including president of the Oklahoma State Dermatological Association

• Publishes regularly in medical journals, including the *Journal of Dermatologic Surgery* and *Dermatologic Surgery and Oncology*

Bernard P. Nusbaum, M.D.
  7867 S.W. 88th Street
  Miami, FL 33156
  (305) 274-2202

• Is a dermatologist (board certified by the American Board of Dermatology)

• Is widely published in fields of dermatology and hair transplantation

• Has published "Hair Transplantation: A Three-Stage Approach for Creating the Hairline," *Journal of Dermatologic Surgery and Oncology* (1992), "Hair Transplantation in Black Patients," *Hair*

Transplant Forum International (1991), and "Frontal Forelock: Overall Design," *Hair Transplant Forum International* (1995).

• Is in demand as a lecturer; has presented dozens of programs, research findings, and clinical reports at medical conferences

• Graduated from the University of Colorado, 1974

• Received doctor of medicine degree from the University of Miami School of Medicine, 1979

• Did internship in internal medicine at Mount Sinai Medical Center, Miami Beach, 1979–1980

• Did residency in dermatology at Mount Sinai, 1980–1983, serving as Chief Resident in Dermatology, 1981–1983

• Has been a Clinical Assistant Professor lecturing in dermatology in the Department of Family Medicine at the University of Miami School of Medicine and has been a clinical instructor at the Department of Dermatology and Cutaneous Surgery at the University of Miami School of Medicine

William R. Rassman, M.D.
    9911 West Pico Blvd.
    Los Angeles, CA 90035
    (310) 553-6790

• Is a surgeon (board certified by the American Board of Surgery)

• With Robert M. Bernstein, M.D., pioneered the follicular transplantation method of hair transplantation (see Chapter Three)

• Received doctor of medicine degree from the Medical College of Virginia, 1966

• Did internship in surgery at the University of Minnesota and later became a cardiac fellow under Dr. C. W. Lillehei

• Did residency in general surgery at Cornell and Dartmouth Medical Centers

• Served in the U.S. Army as a surgeon, 1969–1971; was stationed in Kentucky and in the Republic of Vietnam; was awarded the Silver Star and earned the rank of major

• Conducted major research in the cardiac field and commercialized the Intra-Aortic Balloon Pump in 1969, a device credited today with saving thousands of lives each year; continues to be active in the cardiac field

• Holds patents in numerous fields, from computer software to biotechnology; in the hair transplant field, has pioneered new techniques and invented the Hair Densitometer, which measures hair density and the health of hair

• Is frequently published in medical journals and presents scientific papers before national and international societies

Paul Rose, M.D.
   6140 Bayside Drive
   New Port Richey, FL 34652
   (727) 849-1447

• Is a dermatologist (board certified by the American Board of Dermatology)

• Is Assistant Clinical Professor at the University of South Florida in the Department of Medicine, Division of Dermatology

• Received doctor of medicine degree from the State University of New York at Downstate Medical Center, Brooklyn, New York, 1979

• Did internship in internal medicine at the University of Connecticut Medical Center, Farmington, Connecticut, completed 1980

• Did residency in dermatology at Temple University Skin and Cancer Hospital, Philadelphia, Pennsylvania, completed in 1988

• Has given several presentations on hair restoration to prestigious societies, including a "Live Surgery Workshop for Hair Transplantation" for the American Academy of Cosmetic Surgery

• Has published several articles in the field of micrographic surgery and continues to do research and write in this field

Ron Shapiro, M.D.
    3023 Eastland Blvd., #113
    Clearwater, FL 33761
    (888) 741-1111

• Is an internist (board certified in Internal Medicine)

• Board certified by the American Board of Emergency Medicine

• Graduated from Emory University, 1975

• Received doctor of medicine degree from Emory University School of Medicine, 1979

• Interned in internal medicine at Emanuel Hospital in Portland, Oregon, 1979–1980

• Did residency in internal medicine at Emanuel, 1980–1982

• Was trained in surgical and trauma emergency medicine at Harbor General Hospital, Torrance, California, 1981, and in pediatric emergency medicine at Grady Memorial Hospital, Atlanta, Georgia, 1982

• Is active in professional societies and research and has presented lectures on hair transplantation at medical conferences in the United States and abroad, including live surgery lectures in the United States and Rome

• Has published research papers and articles in medical journals and publications

Bradley R. Wolf, M.D.
  11821 Mason-Montgomery Rd.
  Cincinnati, OH 45249
  (513) 774-0400

• Is a surgeon (board certified in Emergency Medicine)

• Practices exclusively as a transplant surgeon

• Received doctor of medicine degree from Indiana University School of Medicine, 1980

• Did internship in General Surgery at Eastern Virginia Graduate School of Medicine, Norfolk, Virginia, 1980–1981

• Did residency in General Surgery at Eastern Virginia Graduate School of Medicine, Norfolk, Virginia 1981–1982

• Is a member of a number of professional associations

• Has lectured extensively on hair transplantation surgery at medical conferences in the United States, Europe, and Russia

• Has presented live surgery workshops at conferences in the United States and Russia

Essential Oil Treatment

As described in Chapter Two, this basic treatment has been known to trigger hair growth in patients with alopecia areata. Essential oil treatments can also be customized according to type and extent of hair loss, age, and scalp condition. For information regarding a customized formula to treat your hair loss, contact Melanie Von Zabuesnig by fax at (714) 975-3115 or by E-mail at vz@earthlink.net.

Locks of Love

Locks of Love was started in 1997 by Ft. Lauderdale businesswoman Peggy Knight, who lost her hair to alopecia areata at the age of fourteen and is now completely bald. Her nonprofit organization donates wigs to children who have lost their hair due to disease, burns, or cancer treatments.

Custom-made vacuum-fit wigs made from human hair normally retail for about three thousand dollars each. Each uses eight to ten "ponytails" of donated hair. Donated hair must be at least ten inches long and must be washed and dried before cutting. It must be cut as a ponytail or braid and not allowed to drop on the floor. It then must be placed directly in a plastic bag and then a padded envelope for mailing. Permed or dyed hair cannot be accepted.

Locks of Love also accepts monetary donations used to buy synthetic wigs for children with temporary hair loss and to help with office costs such as postage and telephone. All staff members are volunteers. All donations are tax deductible.

If you would like information about receiving a donated wig for a child or are interested in donating, call (888) 896-1588. You can send cut hair to Locks of Love, 1729 E. Commercial Blvd., Suite 207, Ft. Lauderdale, Florida 33334. Ten percent of the hair that's donated comes from children. You can also visit the Locks of Love Web site at www.medicalimage.com/locksoflove.

Index